THE ALCHEMY OF SLEEP

The Science, Mystery & Magic of a Good Night's Rest

DR. PEDRAM NAVAB, FAASM

SHAMBHALA

Shambhala Publications, Inc.
2129 13th Street
Boulder, Colorado 80302
www.shambhala.com

Cover design: Kate E. White
Interior design: Farzana Razak

9 8 7 6 5 4 3 2 1

First Edition
Printed in the United States of America

Shambhala Publications makes every effort to print on acid-free, recycled paper.
Shambhala Publications is distributed worldwide by Penguin Random House, Inc., and its subsidiaries.

LIBRARY OF CONGRESS CATALOGING-IN-PUBLICATION DATA
Names: Navab, Pedram author
Title: The alchemy of sleep: the science, mystery, and magic of a good night's rest / Dr. Pedram Navab.
Description: First edition. | Boulder, Colorado: Shambhala Publications, Inc, [2026] | Includes bibliographical references and index.
Identifiers: LCCN 2026005406 | ISBN 9781645474777 trade paperback
Subjects: LCSH: Sleep | Sleep disorders—Alternative treatment | Mind and body | Mindfulness (Psychology) | Meditation | LCGFT: Popular works
Classification: LCC RA786 .N38 2026
LC record available at https://lccn.loc.gov/2026005406

The authorized representative in the EU for product safety and compliance is eucomply OÜ, Pärnu mnt 139b-14, 11317 Tallinn, Estonia, hello@eucompliancepartner.com.

We all want to dissolve . . .
We all need the experience of forgetting who we are.

AN OLD ZEN MONK QUOTED IN *AFLAME* BY PICO IYER

You wanna fly, you got to give up
the shit that weighs you down.

TONI MORRISON, *SONG OF SOLOMON*

The ultimate act of power is surrender.

KRISHNA DAS

CONTENTS

THE ALCHEMY OF SLEEP

INTRODUCTION

I WAS THIRTY-ONE WHEN SLEEP ALMOST KILLED ME.

Not metaphorically. Not with a tragic burnout story. It tried to end me, literally. It came for me like a fist. Like a wrecking ball of arrogance and blood and metal and speed. Perhaps it came for me because of my lack of regard for it. For the way I had treated it like an afterthought. A weakness. Something other people needed.

I was a neurology resident. I thought I was invincible, that my mind could outrun my body. I thought I could white-knuckle it through anything because I had spent years doing just that. I wore sleeplessness like a badge. Look how far I can push myself! Look what I can survive! Look how close I can get to breaking without actually breaking.

But I finally broke.

It was Labor Day weekend 2002, and I was driving home from Arizona to California. The sky was the kind of endless, driftless blue that makes you forget you're just flesh. I'd been awake for at least thirty hours. I hadn't slept after my shift, telling myself I was fine. Just a little tired. I told myself I could make it because I always made it.

My mind was still in the hospital, replaying labs and seizures and spinal taps; the way the patient's eyes rolled back; the way no one noticed; the things I forgot to write down; the things I couldn't let go of. I wasn't in the car. I was inside my own head, unraveling. What I didn't obsess over—what I barely considered—was my own exhaustion. Sleep, to me, was a limit, an inconvenience, something to be ignored or overcome. I believed I could outwit it, overpower it.

I was wrong.

The desert highway stretched before me, an endless, shimmering ribbon of asphalt. My eyelids grew heavy, fluttering against a relentless wave of drowsiness. I could push through, I told myself. I always had. Just a few more hours, and I'd be home. I don't remember the moment my car veered off the highway. I don't remember the impact, the way metal twisted and crumpled. I don't remember my head striking the car again and again and again. But I do remember the aftermath. I remember gaining consciousness just long enough to taste blood in my mouth. My own. Warm. Metallic. Leaking from my forehead. I remember a distant, phantom voice wailing or screaming or laughing, suggesting, "You've come so far, but this is where the story ends. This is where *you* end."

Then, darkness.

I drifted in and out of consciousness as a helicopter airlifted me to the Intensive Care Unit at The University of Arizona Medical Center in Tucson—the very place where I was training to become a neurologist. (In retrospect, the irony wasn't lost on me.) My injuries were extensive: multiple fractures; lung contusions and pulmonary edema; deep lacerations on my face, body, arms, and legs; and a variety of internal injuries. Months later, long after I had left the hospital, doctors discovered a chronic subdural hematoma—a slow bleed in my brain—that required a craniotomy to drain. I was placed on antiseizure medications that I'm taking to this day. The road to recovery was long and brutal. The physical pain was one thing; the mental and emotional toll was another. I was a doctor treating patients with head trauma while struggling with the lingering effects of my own.

For three months, I stepped away from residency to heal. I needed stillness. I needed what I had spent a portion of my life running from.

I needed sleep.

Not just because I was exhausted, but because I was cracked open. Sleep became the only place I didn't have to try, the only space that asked nothing of me, the only refuge that felt safe. In that stillness, something subtle began to shift—a kind of quiet reassembling that I wouldn't recognize until much later.

I used to treat sleep like a thief. Like something that stole time from me. Now it was the only thing that gave me back time, gave me pieces of myself. That experience changed the trajectory of my life. It led me to pursue a fellowship in sleep medicine at Stanford, where I came to understand what I had ignored for so long: Sleep is not a luxury. It is not expendable. It is fundamental—a biological necessity as crucial as oxygen. My accident was a brutal, unforgiving lesson in what happens when we deny that fact.

Since then, I have dedicated my medical career to educating others about the critical role of sleep. I have served on committees with the American Academy of Sleep Medicine, working to raise awareness of the importance of sleep. I have stood in the halls of Capitol Hill, advocating for policies that acknowledge the life-or-death and debilitating consequences of sleep deprivation.

And yet, as a society, we are still failing. We claim to understand the importance of sleep, but our actions betray us. Schools ring their morning bells before dawn, which leaves children in a chronic state of sleep deprivation. Workplaces glorify long hours over well-rested minds. Medical residencies push doctors past their breaking points, perpetuating the same dangerous myths I once believed. We wear sleep deprivation like a badge of honor, like I once did, mistaking it for strength.

But it's not strength. It's really the body's way of showing how deeply we've forgotten to care for ourselves. The truth is that sleep deprivation isn't just about feeling tired; it's a serious public health hazard. As someone who has spent years studying how sleep shapes the developing brain, I've also worked to bring that science into the real world, most notably by lobbying for later school-start times. It never made sense to me that we expect teenagers, whose biological clocks naturally shift later during adolescence, to perform their best at hours when their brains are still half asleep. I've seen the difference when schools make the change: Students show up more alert, grades rise, and even rates of depression and car accidents drop. It's one of those rare public health interventions that costs almost nothing yet changes everything. Because when kids start school rested instead of running on fumes, we're not just giving them more sleep; we're giving them back their potential.

Research in the medical field reveals public health concerns there too: Residents working extended shifts make 36 percent more serious medical errors and are 61 percent more likely to injure themselves on the job with needle sticks or other accidents.[1] And the risk of a car crash after a night on call? It doubles. Unfortunately, I became one of those statistics. Sleep loss affects everything, from memory to attention to judgment, which are the tools we physicians rely on to save lives. Yet the medical system glorifies endurance over well-being, teaching young doctors to ignore their most basic biological needs. But I can assure you, no patient is safer when their doctor is running on three hours of sleep. And no doctor is invincible. I learned that the hard way.

Like the medical profession, companies have long mistaken exhaustion for work ethic and long hours for productivity. But here's the truth: Sleep-deprived employees make more mistakes, get sick more often, and burn out faster, costing businesses billions. A RAND Corporation study estimated that the United States loses up to $411 billion a year in productivity due to insufficient sleep.[2] That's more than the annual GDP of some countries. And it's not just lost hours. It's poor decision-making, sluggish creativity, and even major errors. Both the Exxon Valdez oil spill and the space shuttle *Challenger* disaster were linked to fatigue. Yet many workplaces still glorify the early-rising, late-working hustle culture. First to work, last to leave becomes a competition. It's shortsighted. A well-rested team is faster, sharper, far more innovative. Imagine a company that treats sleep like it does exercise or mindfulness, not as a luxury but as a tool for peak performance. That shift could change the bottom line—and the culture—entirely.

Sleep-deprived students, doctors, and employees might get through their to-do lists, but they're not the ones who will come up with the next big idea. Creativity thrives in a well-rested brain, one that has had enough REM sleep to connect the dots between seemingly unrelated things, make intuitive leaps, and problem-solve in original ways. When someone is running on fumes, their thinking narrows. They become more reactive than reflective, more task-focused than idea-driven. And that's not the mindset that fuels innovation. If a student wants to excel, a medical office wants to help people, and a company claims to be "visionary" or "future-focused," but they all still expect people to grind through sleepless weeks, they are sabotaging their own goals. Rest isn't the enemy of productivity; it's the secret engine behind every light-bulb moment.

We can do better. We *must* do better. Because when we change the way we sleep, we change everything: our health, our clarity, our very existence. The challenges before us, both personal and planetary, demand our full presence; we can't awaken the world if we ourselves remain half asleep.

EMBRACING SLEEP'S DEEPER MEANING

Although sleep is a necessity, it is much more than that, too. French writer and philosopher Maurice Blanchot said, "There is between sleep and us something like a pact, a treaty with no secret clauses. . . . We surrender to sleep, but in the way that the master entrusts himself to the slave who serves him."[3] Blanchot suggests that sleep isn't something wild or inherently dangerous—it's more like a negotiated truce between us and our need for rest. Like agreeing to a "pact" or "treaty" without any hidden terms, we have come to accept sleep as a necessary and even useful part of our lives. Instead of being overwhelmed or controlled by sleep, we've learned to domesticate it, making it work for us. In this view, surrendering to sleep isn't a sign of weakness but rather a strategic act: Like the tide retreating to gather its strength, we let sleep move through us so that it can restore what the day has spent. This controlled surrender allows sleep to become an instrument that fuels our capacity to act and live effectively, transforming what might seem like vulnerability into a form of strength.

I agree with Blanchot to a point. But his way of thinking has led us down a familiar path—one where we try to hack sleep, track it, and turn it into another form of self-optimization. The truth is simpler and far less technical: Sleep doesn't need decoding; it simply is. Sleep is free, a vital gift that transcends our attempts at control. This more optimistic and modern perspective suggests that sleep's value lies in its spontaneous, liberating nature; it isn't something we command or manage but a natural force that freely renews our bodies and minds. In this view, sleep's gifts are not earned or bargained for; they are simply given, inviting us to partake in a mysterious, regenerative process for our minds and bodies.

Sleep is the one place where we're allowed to disappear without consequences, where the world releases its grip on us, if only we let it. But so many of us fight it. We cling to our thoughts like wreckage in a storm, afraid that if we surrender, we'll lose something vital or miss some elusive answer to a problem that has so far defied resolution. And yet sleep waits for us like a forgiving lover we keep abandoning, forsaking, and dismissing. Sleep is patient, whispering that we don't have to carry it all, we don't have to be it all, we don't have to do it all. For those hours of the night, we can fall, fail, dissolve, be nothing, and still be whole. It's the closest thing we have to mercy, to being held without expectation, to being weightless in a world that is always asking us to bear more, to be more, to feel more, to do more. In a world that can often be cruel, cold, and uncompromising, sleep doesn't want or need anything from us. Yet we resist or suffocate it until exhaustion forces us down like a grieving mother pressing her child to her chest, rocking us into the darkness we should have trusted all along.

Sleep is not an ending to the day but a quiet genesis, a liminal space where we shed what we no longer need. We surrender. We gather the strength to become. It is the pause before creation, where the chaos of waking life retreats. Without sleep, there is no true start: only a continuation, a blurred repetition. Sleep is the first movement, reminding us that to truly begin, we must first let go. Completely. But let go at the proper time, not when you're driving a lonely highway, like I was.

In *How We Live Is How We Die*, the Buddhist teacher Pema Chödrön gently but powerfully returns to the truth of impermanence as something we resist but must eventually embrace.[4] She reminds us that everything—relationships, emotions, even our identity—is in constant flux, and the more we try to hold on, the more we suffer. This has a quiet but profound connection to sleep: Every night, we practice a kind of letting go. We release control, we shed the day's roles, we surrender to the unknown space of dreams and rest. Chödrön's incisive teachings suggest that just as death invites us to release our grip on what we know, so does sleep offer a daily, softer rehearsal for that release. If we can meet impermanence not with fear, but with curiosity or tenderness, our sleep, and even our life, can become more easeful.

At first glance, it might seem as if the title of this book, *The Alchemy of Sleep*, is removed from rest, from a state of recovery, from stillness. Alchemy requires work. It connotes transformation through effort, a drive for mastery, a refinement of skills. It also implies magic and might not seem very practical when discussing sleep, a necessity of life. In many ways, however, *alchemy* is the perfect word for this book because it captures the transformative power of sleep in our lives. Just as ancient alchemists sought to turn base metals into gold, sleep is the natural process by which the mind and body are renewed, stress melts away, and raw experiences are processed into clarity, into wisdom.

While alchemy is often associated with an ancient practice in which the ordinary is metamorphosed into the extraordinary, alchemy transcends such literal meaning to embody the pursuit of spiritual, psychological, and physical transformation that often accompanies restful sleep. When viewed through this lens, alchemy fuses cultural, mystical, and metaphysical perspectives to transform sleep into something that is greater than itself: a renewal, an awakening, a new start. Across many traditions, sleep has been situated in a liminal space—a nightly ritual in which the boundaries between the conscious and unconscious, death and life, dissolve. It is death but not death. It is life but not life. It is death in life. We are somewhere else but not *here*, as we know it. Simultaneously, we are somewhere and nowhere, an uncharted expanse of possibilities. Not here, but not there, either. Our bodies exist, but they exist on a plane that eludes us. We are in a reversible coma, unconscious until we awaken.

From a mystical perspective, sleep is an otherworldly realm for transformation akin to the alchemical process: The soul is finally able to shed the weight of the day, the mind can explore its environs without its daily constraints and obligations, and the body and brain can regenerate. In short, the title of this book reflects how understanding and nurturing sleep can elevate it from a mundane biological need (base metal) to an essential and sacred practice for overall well-being (gold).

But to leave sleep there, in its numinous place, is also not entirely accurate. Notwithstanding its mystical and mythical elements, sleep is also situated in the realm of modern neuroscience. Real, meaningful things, with benefits and consequences, happen there. Tissue regenerates. Memory consolidates. Breathing alters. Debris in the brain is swept away. Housekeeping activities occur.

From a neurological perspective, we have various cast and crew to initiate sleep: The hypothalamus (director) acts as a sleep-wake center, the brainstem (choreographer) maintains wakefulness and transitions between sleep stages, the thalamus (gatekeeper) acts as a relay station for sensory information, the pineal gland (stagehand) regulates circadian rhythms through melatonin production, the cerebral cortex (playwright) processes information and generates dreams, and the amygdala (dramatic actor) manages emotional processing.

Yet, despite these crew and cast members, the theater production, if you will, is not complete. Where is the stage, that backdrop or scenery, which sets the mood for the play? Where is the sound and music that underpins the entire performance and provides the play with that emotional nuance that we can't put into words? Where is the magic that makes a theater production something we'll remember for a long time?

When we marry these two seemingly disparate aspects of sleep, the metaphysical and scientific, it becomes multidimensional: something larger than itself, larger than life. As a neurologist, sleep medicine specialist, and integrative medicine practitioner, my impetus in writing this book is to encourage you to view sleep in both its otherworldly and scientific aspects. I also hope to initiate a dialogue that has been foreclosed for quite some time. Ultimately, I want us to see sleep as an important part of our waking lives—one that enables us to show up and communicate with ourselves and others in a way that is honest, genuine, and meaningful.

Sleep is not a problem to be solved. Instead of engaging in linear thinking, which leads only to finite spaces, we can become more curious about sleep—exploring it and moving it beyond its ordinary, utilitarian role as something we simply need or want, such as food, shelter, or sex. By elevating sleep to a more spiritual plane, we allow ourselves to interact with it, initiate a dialogue, and let it reveal the secrets, darkness, and goodness within us that we often refuse to see. I invite you into that space, with its powerful dreams, shadows, and metaphysical forces—into a vast terrain that is infinitely strange, glorious, unexpected.

It appears to me that a rift has been created between the sciences and the spiritual or mystical aspects of sleep medicine. Neither alone can address sleep and dreams in a way that is genuine, intuitive, productive, or whole. The cast and crew (science) require the set production, music, and creative ingredients of the spiritual and mystical to make the play successful. In part, then, this book was written as an alternative, or at least a counterpart, to the numerous books on sleep hygiene (the healthy habits and environmental factors that promote restful sleep) and cognitive behavioral therapy as a treatment for insomnia (CBT-I), which may address the science and "practical" side of sleep but do not touch on its spiritual and mystical elements. These treatment modalities do not suffice for a large subset of patients who require a more thorough analysis, a deeper understanding of their psyche that has subconsciously created the sleep problems they now face, and integrative practices to work on these deeper levels.

This more modern and intuitive approach to sleep that I use with my patients and outline in this book takes a different trajectory by exploring breathwork, shadow work, and dreamwork, among other techniques, which get to the root of the worrisome thoughts, anxieties, and obsessive thinking that, for a large subset of insomniacs, is the essence of the problem. While traditional sleep medicine, sleep hygiene, and CBT-I have their place, integrative practices reach the hidden undergrowth, the detritus that one can't seem to sweep from the floor. This holistic approach addresses the patient's immediate sleep-related issues and their overall well-being, aiming for sustainable improvements in sleep quality and duration. But it doesn't stop there. It toggles back to science to bring the latest developments from neuroscience into the conversation to see how the two—the science and the mystical—interact and to learn from their synergy.

The Alchemy of Sleep lives at the meeting point of science and spirit. Modern neuroscience can explain what happens in your brain as you drift off, but there's another layer—something mysterious, symbolic, even sacred—that science alone can't capture. In these pages, I invite you to explore both sides: how sleep evolved, how it shapes your mind and body, and how you can use what we now know to rest more deeply. Along the way, you'll find practical tools drawn from both modern medicine and ancient wisdom, ways to quiet the mind, engage with your dreams, and rediscover the wonder of rest. My own years in the sleep clinic have shown me that when these two worlds meet, something extraordinary happens. Sleep becomes more than a biological need; it becomes a teacher, a healer, a mirror for who we are.

Building on what modern brain and sleep research have uncovered, *The Alchemy of Sleep* explores what's happening when you drift off each night: why we need sleep, what goes wrong when we don't get enough, and how common disorders such as insomnia, sleep apnea, and parasomnias can quietly shape our health and moods. But there's another side to sleep that science often overlooks—the mysterious, dream-soaked realm of the subconscious. This is where your mind works through emotions, hunches, and hidden fears, the same forces that can make rest feel so elusive. In this book, we'll wander into that shadow side together. Because when you begin to understand not just how you sleep, but *who* you are in sleep, you start to unlock something powerful: a more peaceful night and a deeper knowing of yourself.

Through simple practices such as shadow work, dream journaling, and breathwork—woven throughout these pages—you'll begin to see how sleep connects you to the deeper parts of yourself that often stay hidden in waking life. This isn't just a book for people who can't sleep; it's for anyone curious about what sleep really means and how it shapes your emotions, your creativity, your sense of self. Here, science meets spirit, helping you understand not only how to rest better but also how to listen to what your dreams and your body are trying to tell you. Sleep isn't just something that happens at night: It's a living conversation between your mind and your soul.

In her short but memorable book *Pause, Rest, Be: Stillness Practices for Courage in Times of Change*, Octavia F. Raheem urges us to "Be still and know. Be still." A restorative yoga practitioner, Raheem considers *savasana*, or the corpse pose, to be the most significant of the yoga poses because it signifies the practice of death. For her, "every ending, big or small, is some kind of death." It is the death of the ego, the death of all aversion to reality. The corpse pose suggests that "for now, there is nothing left to do."[5]

I propose that we situate sleep in this state, too: a zone where we are dead—dead to the world, dead to ourselves—but also where we are at peace to solve problems, grapple with the unknown, and consider possibilities that elude us in the waking world. The voyage of sleep that I outline in this book is a shamanic journey into the heart of the unknown, the heart of light, the heart of darkness, where we simulate death to understand ourselves, our unconscious, better. So, let's begin this glorious expedition into the uncharted unknown, the hinterland, to whatever and wherever it may lead us.

PART ONE

THE SACRED ARCHITECTURE OF SLEEP

1

SLEEP IS YOUR BODY'S SUPERPOWER

IN THIS CHAPTER WE'LL EXPLORE THE SCIENCE OF SLEEP: THE physiology, chemistry, and neural choreography that form the "base metals" of our alchemy. Before we can transform the ordinary into the extraordinary, we must understand what the ordinary is made of. If the scientific parts feel dense or overwhelming, feel free to skip ahead; the spirit of alchemy will still meet you there, in the realms of breath, shadow, and dream.

But first, to understand sleep in all its implications, let's define it physiologically. Sleep is a natural, reversible state of relative inactivity and reduced responsiveness to external stimuli, accompanied by characteristic physiological changes, including decreased sensory perception, muscle relaxation, and a slowed metabolic rate. By contrast, wakefulness is a state of alertness and engagement with the environment. Its characteristics include heightened sensory perception, motor activity, and cognitive functioning. Wakefulness is facilitated by the activity of the reticular activating system (RAS) in the brainstem. Sleep and wakefulness appear to be direct opposites, yet as we'll soon see, they have much in common.

Both states are part of the circadian rhythm that is regulated by the hypothalamic suprachiasmatic nucleus and influenced by external cues of light and darkness. Moreover, virtually all living organisms, including animals, plants, and bacteria, have adapted their physiological parameters to this cycle. The circadian generator in humans is in the suprachiasmatic nucleus (SCN), which lies above (hence, "supra") the crossing point of the optic nerves. Despite being such a small part of the brain, the SCN effectively controls various physiological matters, whether this be our awakenings, sleep schedule, or food consumption. This rhythm is slightly longer than twenty-four hours (on average twenty-four hours and fifteen minutes) and can generate independently of light, although light is a powerful *zeitgeber* ("time giver" in German) and can greatly influence the rhythm in an individual. Melatonin is the signal that connects the SCN to our brain and body, allowing a seamless transition from sleep to wakefulness or from wakefulness to sleep. Its abundance is the signal that it's time for sleep, while its scarcity is the messenger that it's time to wake up.

THE EVOLUTION OF SLEEP

Melatonin's rhythmic rise and fall reminds us that sleep is not simply an optional state of rest, but a deeply conserved biological rhythm woven into our survival. Its orchestration hints at a larger truth: Sleep must serve a purpose far greater than mere restoration. As the prominent sleep researcher Allen Rechtschaffen suggested in 1971, "If sleep does not serve an absolutely vital function, then it is the biggest mistake the evolutionary process has ever made."[1] He highlighted the paradoxical nature of sleep in evolutionary biology and its critical role in survival. In essence, with this statement, Rechtschaffen articulated that sleep seems counterintuitive from an evolutionary standpoint.

For example, during sleep, an organism is inactive, less alert to predators, and unable to perform essential survival functions such as foraging or reproducing. If sleep did not serve a vital function, he suggested, then why did natural selection maintain it and make it so essential to life? Indeed, if sleep were a mistake, it would contradict the efficiency of the evolutionary process, which optimizes traits and behaviors for survival and reproduction. Rechtschaffen's concise statement challenges us to consider why such a seemingly "impractical" state as sleep remains central to survival and well-being. It also provocatively underscores the critical importance of sleep, suggesting that far from being an "evolutionary mistake," it is the cornerstone of health and survival, deeply embedded in the fabric of life.

To better understand why sleep has been so powerfully preserved by evolution, it is useful to consider how human sleep patterns have adapted and diversified throughout our history. By exploring the various ways our ancestors slept, we can gain insight into the vital role that sleep continues to play in our lives today.

Owls and Larks

From the perspective of the circadian rhythm, some of us are "night owls." We prefer to stay awake well into the night and sleep in the early morning hours, naturally waking up in late morning or early afternoon. Others are "early birds," or "morning larks," preferring to go to bed early and rise in early dawn. From an evolutionary perspective, there must have been a reason for this. Considering that early humans cohabitated as families and tribes and often slept together, sleeping at different times was potentially advantageous if they were being hunted by animals or other humans. Essentially, the morning larks would keep watch in the early morning, while the night owls would monitor late into the night.

This "watchful sentinel hypothesis" suggests that while some members were active during the day (the morning larks), others (the night owls) remained alert in the evening and early night, helping to protect the group from predators or threats. From this perspective, nature was resourceful and cunning; it did not make a mistake. In today's world, however, the evolutionary benefits of diverse chronotypes persist in certain contexts, such as shift work or industries that require 24/7 operations. However, the mismatch between chronotype and societal expectations (e.g., early work or school schedules) can lead to circadian misalignment and health issues.

From Branch to Ground

Sleep states during preindustrial times likely included periods of inactivity during the cold seasons and increased activity during the warm seasons. Undoubtedly, once suitable places were made for sleep and to avoid predation, these cycles changed. Because mammals have an enlarged brain compared to other species, some theorists, including the evolutionary biologist J. Lee Kavanau, have suggested that slow-wave and REM sleep developed because these larger brains were able to accommodate the learning, storage, and maintenance of information and memories.

For primitive humans, wakefulness was necessary to sustain attention, learn new information, and to store this data into memory. Sleep, on the other hand, was useful to conserve energy and to avoid the dangers of nocturnal activity. But sleep also made humans (and other mammals) vulnerable to attacks at night and, as such, its evolutionary purpose must have surpassed its inability to be awake to fight predators.

Sleep researchers, such as Frederick L. Coolidge, have argued that *Homo erectus*, which appeared 1.9 million years ago and was a predecessor of *Homo sapiens*, made a full transition from sleeping on branches of trees to sleeping on the ground, which may have had positive cognitive benefits by offering the opportunity for a single uninterrupted sleep period. This provided a survival advantage not only in terms of more restful sleep and energy in battling predators but also through improved cognitive abilities. Ground sleeping also reduced the energy needed to climb trees and maintain balance while sleeping. This saved energy, then, could be redirected toward other survival tasks, such as hunting, foraging, and toolmaking. Moreover, sleeping on the ground also encouraged group cohesion, as individuals needed to rely on one another for protection from predators. This may have fostered the development of stronger social bonds and early forms of cooperation and communication.

Other researchers, such as Matthew Walker, have argued that because sleeping on tree branches was so tenuous and dangerous (especially during REM sleep, when our muscles completely relax and we can potentially fall many feet to the ground), *Homo erectus* was the first biped to sleep completely on the ground, which made sleep more consolidated. But, because of this shift in positions from tree branches to the ground, humans also made themselves prey to insects and large animals. In Walker's opinion, fire and smoke were instrumental in deterring large carnivores and fumigating insects, in turn. Fire not only deterred predators but also created a communal space for groups to gather, socialize, and share knowledge, potentially accelerating the evolution of language and culture. But there remained the possibility of attacks if *Homo erectus* slept longer than was necessary. Here is the real key, though: Sleep for *Homo erectus* became shorter in duration but more packed, especially with REM sleep. Because REM sleep so effectively orchestrates socioemotional signaling, facilitates recognition and comprehension, consolidates memories, and fuels creativity, humans evolved into a cognitive and social powerhouse, forming larger and more complex social groups.[2]

Biphasic Sleep

Recently, there has been an interest in biphasic sleep, referring to a sleep pattern in which a person sleeps in two distinct segments instead of one continuous block. This can take various forms, such as a longer sleep period at night with a shorter nap during the day or, more commonly, a segmented night sleep with a period of wakefulness in between. Historically, before the advent of artificial lighting, particularly before the Industrial Revolution, biphasic sleep was the norm in many societies, which we may have difficulty understanding in our society obsessed with a full night of sleep. Historical records, including texts from the Middle Ages and early modern Europe, describe a pattern where people would go to sleep shortly after dusk, wake up for an hour or two in the middle of the night (often engaging in reading, prayer, quiet socializing, or sex), and then return to sleep for a second phase until morning. This pattern, sometimes called "first sleep" and "second sleep," is discussed and documented by the historian A. Roger Ekirch in his book *At Day's Close: Night in Times Past,* where he found references to this natural sleep rhythm in literature, scientific texts, and personal diaries.[3]

Some researchers speculate that sleep-maintenance insomnia—a condition where people wake up in the middle of the night and struggle to return to sleep—may be a remnant of this historically normal biphasic sleep pattern. The idea is that our biological clock may still be wired for segmented sleep, but modern schedules and artificial lighting suppress it.

The idea of biphasic sleep—sleeping in two separate periods during the night—is interesting. I mention it not just to explain a possible evolutionary reason for why people sometimes wake up in the middle of the night, but also to help ease anxiety about this experience. Many people, including some of my patients, worry that waking up at night means something is wrong with them. In reality, our brains might naturally be wired this way.

Learning about the historical basis for biphasic sleep can help reduce worries about disrupted sleep. It can also encourage people to see this pattern as normal rather than a problem. Realizing that sleep is different for everyone, and that waking up at night might be completely natural for some people, can help us accept and adapt to our own sleep patterns. Waking up in the middle of the night isn't dangerous or a sign of poor health—it's just one way that sleep can work.

AN ATLAS OF THE SLEEPING MIND

Every night, your brain moves through a precise sequence of stages, like a silent choreography meant to restore you. Once you understand this process, you start to see why sleep isn't a luxury or a mystery; it's the most important thing you do without trying. Sleep is divided into two major categories: non-rapid eye movement sleep (NREM) and rapid eye movement sleep (REM). A full sleep cycle typically lasts 90 to 120 minutes and repeats four to six times per night. It begins in NREM sleep, which has three stages, and then progresses to REM. The proportion of REM sleep increases in later cycles, while deep NREM sleep dominates earlier cycles.

NREM Sleep

Stage one of NREM sleep (N1) is the light sleep that characterizes the transition from wakefulness to sleep. Theta waves, which have slow, gentle rhythms of 4 to 7 Hz, replace alpha waves, which have a rhythm of 8 to 13 Hz and are the predominant waves during wakefulness. (On an EEG, your brain's activity appears as waves: ripples of electricity moving across your mind. Their speed, measured in hertz, tells the story of your inner state: quick, lively waves when you're awake; slower, rolling ones as you drift into deeper sleep.) Theta waves help your brain disengage from the sensory input of the outside world. It's like your brain is "idling," preparing to dive deeper into sleep, but it's not quite there yet. The duration of this stage is mere minutes, comprising 5 to 10 percent of total sleep time. You can be easily awakened from sleep at this stage, especially by sensations such as falling or abrupt muscle contractions, which are referred to as hypnic jerks. In fact, there is a theory that the hypnic or hypnagogic jerk, which occurs in nearly all primates, might be an archaic remnant to signal that the primate is falling out of the tree. It may have allowed the sleeper to adjust their sleeping position in a nest or on a branch to prevent a fall.[4]

Stage two of NREM sleep (N2) is a continuation of light sleep and accounts for 50 to 55 percent of total sleep time. In this stage, the brain settles into a rhythm. Body temperature drops, heart rate slows, and you become less aware of your surroundings. Bursts of rapid brain activity (12 to 16 Hz) called sleep spindles appear and are thought to protect you from external disruptions (like noise) and help with memory consolidation. K-complexes, sudden large brain waves, further characterize this stage. These complexes help with transitioning into deeper sleep and processing information from the day.

Stage three of NREM sleep (N3), also known as deep sleep or slow-wave sleep, comes next. It's the most restorative stage of NREM sleep, dominated by delta waves (slow, high-amplitude waves of 0.5 to 4 Hz). When delta waves are present, your brain is repairing and recharging. This stage comprises 20 to 25 percent of total sleep time, occurring more in the first half of the night. It's the deepest and most rejuvenating phase of sleep. If someone wakes you up during this stage, you will be groggy and experience sleep inertia, meaning you'll have difficulty acclimating to your environment right away. This stage is also critical for physical recovery, immune function, and memory consolidation, helping to strengthen and solidify newly learned facts, events, and personal experiences so you can recall them later. It is also when pruning (the process of removing unnecessary connections, or synapses, between brain cells) occurs. If you have somnambulism (sleepwalking), night terrors, or confusional arousals, they take place in this stage.

We do dream during non-REM sleep, but these dreams are usually less vivid and more like everyday thoughts or concerns. They tend to be realistic, brief, and lack the strong emotions or detailed stories found in REM dreams.

REM Sleep

REM sleep, perhaps the most studied and enigmatic stage, comprises the last stage of sleep. During this stage, the EEG waves are mixed frequency (fast, low-amplitude waves) and resemble the brain's activity when awake. Like stage three NREM, it comprises 20 to 25 percent of total sleep time. REM sleep becomes more frequent and increases in duration as the night progresses. This stage is often called "paradoxical sleep" because it exhibits a unique combination of both deep sleep and wake-like brain activity. Your brain is highly active, yet your body remains in a state of profound muscle atony, or paralysis, to prevent you from acting out your dreams. Your body is experiencing two opposing physiological states: heightened cortical activity, rapid eye movements, and irregular breathing and heart rate contrasted with near-total muscle inhibition. Additionally, REM sleep is when you have vivid, bizarre dreams, making it an even more fascinating and complex mystery.

In this stage of sleep, your eyes also dart rapidly under your closed eyelids. Because your eye muscles are controlled higher in the brain stem—unlike your facial and skeletal muscles—they're free to move quickly, hence the term "rapid eye movement." Since your eyes aren't involved in moving your body or waking you up, they are immune to the muscle paralysis that keeps the rest of you still. This stage of sleep is vital for emotional regulation, learning, and memory. In fact, when your brain is developing in the womb, about 90 percent of your sleep is spent in the dream-filled REM stage—much higher than the 20 to 25 percent REM sleep you get as an adult.

The particular kind of memory that your brain is processing in REM sleep is procedural memory, especially for activities that require learning motor skills, such as playing an instrument or riding a bike. John Allan Hobson, an eminent dream researcher, even suggested that the maintenance function theory of dreams is viable perhaps because we are rehearsing basic motor skills specific to the tasks that we are undertaking.[5] In this sense, the acquisition of procedural memory in REM sleep makes sense. As a result, obtaining adequate REM sleep can significantly solidify that memory and improve our performance in the task at hand. Meaning if you want to get better at something, you'll need to sleep long enough to experience REM sleep.

REM sleep is also when your brain gets weird, in the best possible way. It's the dream stage where your thoughts loosen up, allowing your mind to jump between unrelated ideas and make surprising connections. That's one reason why REM is such a gold mine for creativity. One study showed that people were better at solving creative problems after REM sleep compared to other stages.[6] The brain's chemistry during REM—which is low in stress chemicals such as norepinephrine—lets you think more freely and abstractly. Dream logic helps us connect the dots in ways our waking minds wouldn't dare. Because REM sleep gets longer throughout the night and into early morning, you're likely to wake in REM sleep, having dreamed or remembering your dreams.

Salvador Dalí was known for tapping into the magic of the wild mind in REM sleep. But he didn't just wait for REM sleep—he hunted it. To access the surreal imagery of his dreams, he used a clever trick: He'd sit in a chair holding a key over a metal plate as he drifted off. Just as he entered the edge of REM sleep, his muscles would relax (due to the muscle paralysis in this stage of sleep), the key would fall, and the clang would wake him, catching him mid-dream. He called this technique "slumber with a key," and it gave him direct access to the bizarre, dreamlike visions that defined his art. For Dalí, REM wasn't just rest; it was inspiration, and his surrealistic artwork reflects the fantastical nature of our dreams.

While it's known as the stage for vivid dreams, REM sleep is also pivotal for processing emotions and refining our ability to interpret facial expressions. Research indicates that REM sleep significantly enhances our capacity to recognize and remember emotional facial expressions. One study demonstrated that individuals who experienced more REM sleep showed improved speed and accuracy in identifying emotional expressions the following day. This suggests that REM sleep facilitates the consolidation of emotional memories, particularly those related to facial cues.[7]

Conversely, lack of REM sleep can impair your emotional acuity. A study used fMRI scans to show that sleep-deprived individuals had heightened amygdala activity and impaired prefrontal regulation when viewing expressive faces. As a result, they were more likely to interpret neutral or ambiguous expressions as threatening. These findings underscore the idea that REM sleep isn't just restorative for the body; it's also essential for our social survival. Being well rested makes us more perceptive, more attuned to others' emotions, and less likely to misread a frown as a threat.[8] I'm sure you've experienced this in real life when you haven't obtained enough sleep. A simple smile could be construed as indifference, no smile as hostility.

Perhaps one of the most interesting aspects of REM sleep is the way it prevents you from acting out your dreams. In one seminal study, scientists found that when the brain cells that normally keep muscles still during REM sleep were damaged, cats started to physically act out their dreams—jumping, clawing, even attacking invisible prey.[9] REM sleep is so vital that when it's taken away, the brain pushes back, flooding you with even more of it the next time you sleep. Some sleep scientists call REM sleep a third state of consciousness, much like ancient

Hindu texts that describe waking (*vaiswanara*), deep sleep (*prajna*), and dream sleep (*taijasa*) as separate levels of awareness.[10]

Cycles of Creation and Destruction

When the normal sleep stages are "balanced," your sleep has a cyclical nature that alternates between destruction and creation, with each cycle replaying every ninety minutes, and REM sleep becoming lengthier and more frequent throughout the night. NREM removes the neural connections that are no longer necessary, while REM strengthens connections that are vital for memory consolidation. Each cycle of NREM and REM builds upon the last to ensure that your brain and body remain functional and adaptable, reflecting the natural rhythms of creation and destruction in life.

You can think of slow-wave sleep (NREM) as the destruction phase of sleep, clearing out the metabolic waste products of the brain through the *glymphatic* system (more on this later), as well as eliminating weaker or unnecessary neural connections, which is crucial for brain efficiency. On the other hand, REM sleep plays a creative role, contributing to the development of neural networks that fosters creativity and insight through the synthesis of disparate pieces of information (often experienced as dreams). This duality of destruction and creation mirrors the broader natural and universal cycles, such as the death of old cells making way for new growth.

In both Buddhist and Hindu traditions, the concept of samsara represents the continuous cycle of creation, destruction, and rebirth. The daily sleep cycle can be seen as a microcosm of samsara, where the destruction (clearing during NREM) parallels death, and the creation (learning and renewal during REM) parallels rebirth. From this perspective, then, each sleep cycle reflects the impermanence of the day's experiences, which are transformed during the night into new states (e.g., processed memories, refreshed body).

In both the Buddhist and Hindu traditions, however, the goal is liberation (moksha in Hinduism, nirvana in Buddhism) from the repetitive cycle of samsara. Just as spiritual liberation involves transcending cycles of creation and destruction, deep slow-wave sleep symbolizes a temporary liberation, a state of renewal beyond the chaos of daily life.

THE BIOLOGY OF SLEEP REGULATION

When it comes to getting good sleep, two major biological processes work behind the scenes: process C (circadian rhythm) and process S (sleep drive). Returning to the film analogy, you can think of these two as the producers that ensure that the film has funding and production is on track. These two systems work together—one controlling when you feel awake and the other building up your need for sleep. When they're in sync, you sleep well. When they're out of balance, that's when sleep problems begin.

Process C is your circadian rhythm, the internal clock in your brain that runs on roughly a twenty-four-hour cycle. It's controlled by the suprachiasmatic nucleus (SCN) in the hypothalamus, which responds to light and darkness. In the morning, light from the sun (if you happen to be outside) enters your eyes, signaling your brain to stop producing melatonin, the hormone that makes you sleepy. Your body temperature rises, and alertness kicks in. As the sun sets, melatonin levels start increasing, preparing your body for sleep. At night, melatonin peaks, your body temperature drops, and you become naturally drowsy. Process C is important because if your circadian rhythm is off—from jet lag, night shifts, or too much screen time at night—you might wake up at odd hours or struggle to fall asleep. In these instances, your circadian rhythm has been misaligned and skewed. Because of these two processes, and for restful sleep in general, you should awaken at the same time each morning. Waking up at 8:00 a.m. one day and 11:00 a.m. the next will put your body in a state of jet lag, as if you were flying over different time zones. It's one of the simplest things you can do to align your circadian rhythm and ensure restful sleep. Consistency is key.

It's important to understand that your circadian rhythm is shaped by both genetics and external factors such as light and melatonin. These external cues are called *zeitgebers* ("time-givers") because they help set the timing of your internal clock. Your metabolism is closely linked to your circadian rhythm, influencing when you eat and when your body produces chemicals such as cortisol. The field of *chronomedicine* has emerged from this understanding and may one day help determine the best times to take medications for maximum effectiveness.

While your circadian rhythm controls when you should sleep, process S (sleep drive) controls how much sleep you need. Think of it like a sleep pressure meter. The longer you're awake, the more adenosine (a sleep-inducing chemical) builds up in your brain. The more adenosine you accumulate, the sleepier you feel. You can also think of adenosine as a natural anesthetic agent: Once it reaches a critical threshold, you will fall asleep. As you sleep, adenosine is cleared out and you start the process again. Caffeine blocks adenosine receptors, which is why it keeps you awake even when you should be tired. If you take long naps and drink caffeine too late, your sleep pressure may not be strong enough at bedtime, making it difficult to fall asleep. Interestingly, caffeine only blocks adenosine receptors and does not eliminate them. Because of this, once that caffeine is eliminated from the bloodstream, the accumulated adenosine is still there, causing an unanticipated crash of exhaustion. That's why caffeine is not the best solution to sleepiness, because it wreaks havoc on your circadian system and hinders the consistency that is key to good sleep.

Your best sleep happens when both your sleep drive (process S) and your circadian rhythm (process C) are in sync. When your sleep drive is high and your circadian rhythm signals it's time for bed, you'll fall asleep easily and rest well. But if one system is out of sync—such as staying up late despite feeling tired or trying to sleep at an unusual time—your sleep quality will suffer. Ideally, your circadian rhythm boosts alertness and cortisol in the morning, dips in the afternoon, and then gradually winds down in the evening. Meanwhile, your sleep drive steadily increases throughout the day. When these natural rhythms work together, they set the stage for healthy, restorative sleep.

While we can track the physiological processes that constitute the circadian rhythm, these cycles aren't understood solely through biology; they echo an older understanding found in wisdom traditions (particularly Buddhism and Hinduism), where balance and cyclical motion are seen as the essence of life itself: waking and sleeping, expansion and return, the constant flow between two poles that sustain us. Just as yin and yang in Eastern philosophy represent opposing yet complementary forces, process C and process S work in harmony to regulate sleep. In Hinduism, for example, the cycle of creation, preservation, and dissolution (Brahma, Vishnu, Shiva) mirrors how wakefulness builds energy, sleep restores it, and dreams dissolve mental clutter.

Buddhism's emphasis on impermanence (*anicca*), too, reflects how sleep is not a static state but a dynamic flow between wakefulness and rest, dictated by these two processes. When these systems are aligned, we experience deep, restorative sleep, just as spiritual enlightenment comes from harmony with our natural rhythms. Disruptions to this balance, whether in sleep or in life, lead to suffering, whether through insomnia, restlessness, or mental agitation, much like attachment and craving disrupt inner peace. We can now see that aligning our sleep with natural cycles is not just biological but also a spiritual practice, a way of surrendering to the ebb and flow of existence. We can look beyond the science to discover alternative ways of understanding ourselves and the mysteries of sleep, which we'll do more in part two of this book.

THE BENEFITS OF SLEEP

Sleep is not a passive state of rest but an active, highly orchestrated biological process that supports nearly every system in the body. In the sections that follow, we will explore six core benefits of sleep: energy conservation, memory consolidation, cardiovascular health and neural housekeeping, physical and cognitive recovery, immune resilience, and the restoration of inner balance. Together, these processes reveal why sleep is foundational not only to survival but also to vitality and meaning.

Energy Conservation

Sleep serves numerous functions, many of which have been clearly outlined by science and some that have not yet been articulated. Sleep researchers, however, can agree on the most practical and conspicuous purpose: energy conservation. When we sleep, we reduce our energy demands, which is important because we only have a finite amount of energy to meet the demands of being alive. From an evolutionary perspective, this is especially significant. Consider mammals such as sharks and porpoises that have relatively large brains for their body size. These animals have developed unique strategies to conserve energy—porpoises, for example, sleep with one hemisphere of their brain at a time, alternating every fifteen minutes so they can continue to swim and remain alert to danger. Interestingly, REM sleep requires more energy than other stages of sleep, suggesting that despite its high energy cost, it offers important evolutionary benefits that make it essential to survival.

Memory Consolidation

Consolidation of memory and better recall have also been touted as a significant benefit of sleep. Numerous studies have illustrated that memory after having slept is better than after wakefulness. It appears that sleep eliminates irrelevant memory from storage to allow more pertinent information to be stored and recalled. As previously mentioned, slow-wave sleep solidifies declarative memory (what can be recalled, facts, textbook-like memory), while REM sleep bolsters procedural memory (visual and motor skill learning, such as playing an instrument or riding a bicycle). Furthermore, memory that is emotionally charged (celebratory or traumatic events) will have a better chance of consolidation into long-term memory.

As we move through the stages of sleep, the brain begins sorting the day's experiences, deciding what to keep and what to let go. The hippocampus is like our brain's temporary memory desk. It's a small, seahorse-shaped region tucked away in your medial temporal lobe that helps us form new short-term memories. Think of it as the place where our brain first files away bits of information from our day. Then, when we sleep, especially during deep sleep and REM, the hippocampus gets to work replaying those experiences, almost like reviewing our notes. This replay helps transfer the memories to the cortex, which acts as our long-term storage system, keeping them safe and accessible for the future. Interestingly, after this transfer of memory, subsequent sleep allows these files to be "saved." In short, without sleep, our brain's "file transfer" from short-term to long-term memory and "save" function wouldn't work nearly as well.[11]

Sleep has also been hypothesized to strengthen the synapses, or connections between neurons, which are placed under stress during wakefulness when learning occurs. It appears that the rejuvenation sleep affords allows these synapses to strengthen again so that new learning can occur. This hypothesis is bolstered by the fact that sleep in infants and young children has the greatest percentage of REM sleep when such neural strengthening is necessary.[12]

Heart Health and Housekeeping in the Brain

Sleep is also one of the most powerful ways our body protects our heart and brain. While we sleep, our blood pressure naturally dips, our heart rate slows down, and our body releases hormones that reduce inflammation and repair blood vessels. This nightly "reset" helps lower our risk of cardiovascular events such as heart attacks and strokes. Chronic sleep deprivation, on the other hand, keeps our nervous system revved up, raises blood pressure, increases cortisol (the stress hormone), and can trigger irregular heart rhythms. Over time, this stress load adds up, damaging our heart and increasing the chances of a stroke.

When we throw daylight saving time into the mix, things get more problematic. That one-hour shift in the spring, when we "lose" an hour of sleep, may seem harmless, but studies show a noticeable spike in heart attacks and strokes in the days that follow. Why? That sudden change disrupts our circadian rhythm, essentially throwing off the internal clock that regulates everything from blood pressure to blood clotting. Even small amounts of sleep loss or rhythm disruption can act like a mini shock to the system, especially in people already at risk. It's a fascinating and alarming reminder that our body runs on rhythm, and messing with it even a little can have big consequences.

The same principle applies when we travel across time zones. Jet lag is, in a sense, daylight saving time magnified. It's an internal tug-of-war between the body's clock and the sun's clock. Until the brain's circadian rhythm catches up, every system feels slightly off balance: Sleep becomes fragmented, hormones misfire, and even the heart's rhythm can lose its usual steadiness.

As a neurology resident, I dreaded the week after daylight saving time. Every year, like clockwork, our stroke census would increase. The first couple of times I thought it was just a coincidence. But by year three, I started bracing for it like a mini disaster drill. More pages.

More code strokes. More families in shock, asking how their healthy loved one could collapse just getting out of bed. Sleep isn't just a luxury; it's like neurological armor. And when we mess with the clock, the brain keeps the receipts.

Many studies have shown that sleep appears to be the main conduit by which metabolites, or a cell's waste products, are cleared by the brain. During sleep, the brain undergoes such crucial housekeeping processes, which are facilitated by the glymphatic system, flushing out toxins such as amyloid beta and tau proteins—substances linked to the development of Alzheimer's disease. If sleep is consistently disrupted or insufficient, these waste products can accumulate in the brain, creating an environment conducive to neurodegeneration. Chronic sleep deprivation has been strongly associated with increased amyloid beta deposition, a hallmark of Alzheimer's, highlighting the significance of restorative sleep in maintaining brain health and reducing the risk of cognitive decline.

Insufficient sleep sets off a cascade of events in the brain that may contribute to Alzheimer's disease. During sleep, especially deep, restorative sleep, the glymphatic system acts as a sort of nightly cleaning crew, flushing out metabolic waste including amyloid beta, a protein that can clump together to form amyloid plaques. Over time, when we don't get enough sleep, this clearance process is less effective, allowing amyloid to accumulate. Meanwhile, chronic sleep loss also affects the hippocampus, the brain's memory center, making it more vulnerable to damage and impairing the very processes that help consolidate new memories. Together, these factors create an environment where Alzheimer's pathology can take root and progress.

Think of your brain as a busy office building that generates waste throughout the day. Sleep is the night shift that comes in to remove all the trash. If that cleaning crew doesn't show up regularly, the garbage starts piling up, like how insufficient sleep can lead to a buildup of amyloid plaques and other harmful proteins. While some famous historical figures, such as Leonardo da Vinci and Nikola Tesla, were reputed to function on very little sleep, and although they are often mythologized for their sleepless lifestyles, modern research warns that chronic sleep deprivation in our everyday lives is linked to increased Alzheimer's risk. Quality sleep is crucial to keeping our brain "office" clean and our memory center (the hippocampus) in top shape.

Physical and Cognitive Recovery

Adequate sleep is a powerhouse for athletes and anyone looking to optimize their physical performance, too. When we catch enough quality sleep, our body releases growth hormone—crucial for repairing muscle tissues and building strength after intense workouts. Think of it as your body's nightly maintenance crew: It reduces inflammation, helps prevent injuries, and even sharpens your reaction times by consolidating motor skills learned during practice. For example, many professional athletes incorporate specific sleep routines into their training, finding that a consistent seven to nine hours of sleep not only speeds up recovery but also gives them that extra edge in performance when it comes to precision and endurance.[13]

Sleep also plays a significant role in stroke recovery. After a stroke, the brain reconfigures neural pathways to compensate for lost functions. Quality sleep supports this process by enhancing memory consolidation and cognitive repair, effectively giving the brain time to rewire itself. For instance, stroke survivors who maintain regular sleep patterns often report better improvements in language and motor skills during rehabilitation.[14] In both athletic performance and medical recovery, then, sleep isn't just about feeling rested; it's a critical component of the healing and improvement process, acting as a natural enhancer for physical and cognitive functions.

Sleep also directly affects how we feel and process pain. Restful sleep increases our pain threshold, meaning it takes more pain for us to feel it; restless sleep or lack of sleep decreases it, and we feel more pain than we should. As you can see, this becomes a vicious cycle. When you're in pain, you cannot sleep; and when you cannot sleep, your pain level becomes greater. Obviously, you will need to address the pain. But, just as important, your sleep needs a re-working. Ensure that you're obtaining adequate hours of sleep so that you can mitigate your pain level.

Boosting Your Immune System

In this age of emerging viruses of all kinds (avian flu, the novel coronavirus, influenza, etc.), it's important to realize that sleep plays a critical role in supporting the immune system. Sleep promotes the production of immune cells and antibodies. Studies have shown that people who obtain adequate sleep before and after a vaccination produce more robust levels of antibodies compared to those who are sleep deprived. A study on the hepatitis B vaccine found that individuals who had better sleep in the nights following vaccination had nearly twice the antibody response as those with insufficient sleep.[15] Research on the flu vaccine similarly showed that sleep-deprived individuals developed weaker immune responses.[16] During deep sleep, our immune system gets to work, releasing proteins called cytokines that help us battle inflammation and infection. One fascinating study really drove this point home: Researchers found that people who slept less than seven hours a night were almost three times more likely to catch a cold after being exposed to the virus than those who obtained eight hours or more.[17] All these examples suggest that insufficient sleep affects the type of response that individuals have to vaccines. To sleep better is to fight all these viruses better.

Other immunological elements that adequate sleep promotes include more robust levels of T cells, cytokine production, and memory cells.

T cells, which are crucial for identifying and attacking infected cells, function better when you are well rested. Sleep deprivation has been shown to reduce T cell activity, potentially impairing immune defense. Similarly, during slow-wave sleep, the body releases cytokines—proteins that help regulate immunity, inflammation, and responses to infection. Chronic sleep deprivation can reduce the production of these protective cytokines, weakening the immune system over time. Moreover, sleep helps the immune system "remember" antigens, those foreign invaders that attempt to evade us, encountered during vaccination or infection. This process is critical for developing long-lasting immunity.

Restoring Your Inner Balance

There are days when everything just seems a little more overwhelming and taxing than it should. Despite your poor sleep, you had great intentions and a positive demeanor when you woke up, but everything just goes to shit: You hit the alarm's snooze button too hard, which makes the bottle of water on your nightstand fall and spill on the floor; when you stand to clean the floor, you slip and hurt your back. Because you're in so much pain, you get back into bed, calling in sick to work. The day is wasted. Your frustration escalates. You're curt with everyone you speak to. Even your favorite coffee doesn't seem to fix your mood. You realize that sleep had something to do with this mess that you find yourself in. It's no surprise, then, that the relationship between who we are in our daily lives—our mood, health, energy, even how we interact with others—and the quality of our sleep is as intricate as it is important. Think of it as the ultimate feedback loop: Your sleep affects your life, and your life affects your sleep, and your sleep affects your life. And on it goes.

Sleep sets the tone for your mood. The phrase "waking up on the wrong side of the bed" is not just a figure of speech. Sleep and mood are deeply intertwined. A poor night's sleep doesn't just make us feel tired: It lowers our tolerance for stress, heightens emotional reactivity, and clouds our ability to see the brighter side of things. It's like taking life annoyances and turning up the volume. In the scenario above, if we had had a good night's sleep, perhaps we could've looked at things differently, more optimistically. We could've been grateful that we didn't strike our head and cause a bleed in our head when we slipped on the floor, that our boss was understanding of our situation, and that we had the luxury of staying in bed to nurse the pain in our lower back. But we chose the dark side of things, and our pessimism, irritability, and frustration grew proportionally.

On the flip side, good sleep acts like a reset button for our brain. During deep sleep, our brain processes emotions, filing away what's worth remembering and letting go of what's not. Sleep acts as a tabula rasa, a blank slate, allowing us to start anew and fresh. After a restorative night, we wake up feeling more even-keeled, more patient, and even a little more optimistic. We view people, things, and events differently and more joyfully. We begin to love life, or at the least, appreciate life. This is the life that we want to experience daily. And good, restful sleep makes this possible.

Think of your body as a factory of sorts, running its most critical maintenance during sleep. When you skimp on sleep, it's like skipping the repair schedule. It doesn't take long before things start breaking down. When I don't sleep well, I can feel my mind start to unravel, and I know I'm not alone. Everything gets louder: worries, doubts, and small irritations suddenly feel huge. That's what sleep does quietly each night; it pulls us back into balance. It helps us reset, steady our emotions, and see things clearly again. Sleep doesn't just restore the body; it restores who we are when we feel most like ourselves.

We have all noticed how much more difficult it is to deal with people when we're running on fumes, when we can't be bothered to speak to anyone. We may feel guilty about it, but we tell ourselves that it's not our problem to deal with. We blame it on sleep, or the lack thereof, without realizing that the problem resides with us and the framework that we have chosen to deal with our daily scenarios and interactions. Sleep deprivation impairs the prefrontal cortex, the part of our brain responsible for decision-making and impulse control. It also adversely disrupts the amygdala, the emotional control center. As a result, we're more irritable, less empathetic, and prone to snapping at someone over something trivial. Restful sleep, however, does the opposite. It boosts our ability to connect with others, properly read social cues, and respond thoughtfully and appropriately. In other words, sleep makes us a better friend, partner, parent, and co-worker.

A vicious cycle ensues during the stress/sleep tug-of-war. Stress affects your sleep, and poor sleep makes us more stressed. Individuals who are sleep-deprived perceive the world as more stressful because their threshold for stress has been lowered. It doesn't take much, then, for that stress to reveal itself. When life feels overwhelming, your brain is like a car stuck in overdrive: The car's engine is running at a lower rpm but drives at a higher speed and keeps running and running. Because stress can cause insomnia and insomnia can worsen stress, you have two opportunities to mitigate the damage. You can lower your stress level (through meditation, yoga, and so forth), which will improve your sleep. Or you can work on your sleep, which will improve your stress. Two modes of attack are available to you.

Even when you're exhausted, your mind refuses to hit the brakes. Racing thoughts, tension, and a restless body make sleep feel impossible. Despite these detriments, sleep is also one of the best stress relievers. During REM sleep, your brain works through emotional challenges, almost like therapy. It's the reason that restful sleep can make yesterday's problems feel just a little more manageable.

So, how do you escape the push-pull of sleep and life? How do you allow yourself to benefit from sleep at its fullest? How do you let go and allow sleep to do its thing? The key is to view sleep not as a luxury but as a foundation. Begin with small changes: create a bedtime routine, limit screen time before bed, and prioritize winding down even on your busiest days. These habits signal to our body and mind that it's safe to shift gears to a slower speed, to allow the car to eventually come to a halt. This is no overdrive. It's a full stop. Equally important, pay attention to how your daytime choices affect your nights. Are you staying active, eating well, and managing stress? Are you giving yourself permission to rest, or are you wearing exhaustion as a badge of honor—"I'll sleep when I'm dead"?

THE MYTH OF "CATCHING UP" ON SLEEP

We try to hoard hours the way misers hoard coins, hoping that sleeping in on Sunday morning can buy back what Monday through Saturday stole. But let's make this clear: Sleep debt cannot ever be repaid. The idea of "catching up on sleep" sounds comforting, like we can just make a deposit into our sleep bank over the weekend and all will be forgiven. But sleep doesn't work like a savings account. Once we lose deep, quality sleep, we can't fully make it up. Sure, our body might let us sleep in a bit longer after a rough night, but we're not getting back everything that was lost, especially when it comes to all the benefits we've just reviewed, such as memory consolidation, immune function, and emotional regulation.

Think of it like this: Imagine you spend three nights only sleeping four hours each night because you're cramming for an exam or finishing a project. Then, on Saturday, you sleep for ten hours straight. You'll feel a little better, no doubt—more alert, maybe less grumpy. But your brain doesn't just recreate the REM cycles or deep slow-wave sleep it missed earlier in the week. Those opportunities are gone. Studies show that while there might be a brief rebound in deep sleep, it's never enough to fully restore what was lost. Chronic sleep debt, even in small amounts, adds up. Over time, it affects everything from blood sugar levels and cognitive performance to mood and cardiovascular health.

In essence, sleep isn't a commodity we can hoard or restore at will. It's a daily biological need, such as eating or breathing. Miss it, and you don't just get tired: You function differently. That's the reason why consistent, high-quality sleep is far more powerful than binge-resting. Your brain loves rhythm. And when you respect that rhythm, it pays you back in clarity, energy, and resilience.

Sleep, then, is more than just something we do at night, something that we need to "get by." It's magical. It's extraordinary, if we really think about it. It's a reflection of how we live, think, feel. Who we are during the day shapes our sleep, and our sleep shapes who we are during the day. It's the most important and significant relationship that we can nurture because when we take care of our sleep, we're really taking care of ourselves: It's an investment in our tomorrow. As Octavia F. Raheem suggests in her book *Rest Is Sacred,* "To lie down is power, a place to fall apart and be knit back together. Come here and be undone."[18] Sleep is such a cycle, a continuum of falling apart and coming together, of disintegration and consolidation. We must not be afraid of sleep because the process of letting go is what enables us to become who we were meant to be, learning from our shadows and dreams, from the unconscious that we have repressed in our waking lives.

The science of sleep gives us the framework—the how and why—but it can only take us so far. Facts may explain the stages, the rhythms, and the brain waves, but they cannot capture what it feels like to surrender to sleep. To understand that, we must dive deeper. We must go beneath the data, into the quieter, more mysterious territory where science meets the soul. But first, let's turn to what sleep does for our brain and psychological health.

2

HOW SLEEP UNLOCKS YOUR BRAIN'S POTENTIAL

SLEEP IS FAR MORE THAN JUST A NIGHTLY PAUSE; IT'S A DYNAMIC, carefully coordinated process that draws on a symphony of brain chemicals and hormones. Understanding the science behind how we fall asleep, stay asleep, and wake refreshed reveals just how intricate—and essential—this nightly ritual is.

THE ROLE OF NEUROTRANSMITTERS AND HORMONES IN SLEEP

By the time evening arrives, your brain has already been working behind the scenes, preparing for the night ahead. As light fades, the suprachiasmatic nucleus—the brain's internal timekeeper—gets the message that it's time to shift gears. It releases more melatonin, drops your body temperature, and mutes the chatter of neurotransmitters that keep you awake, allowing you to feel the slower rhythms of GABA (gamma-aminobutyric acid) and adenosine. This isn't a passive shutdown but a precise, orchestrated transition; it's a handoff between systems that have spent all day gathering, sorting, and reacting to the world.

When this system works as intended, sleep unlocks the brain's greatest superpower: its ability to learn, adapt, and reinvent itself. During deep sleep, the balance of neurotransmitters shifts: Serotonin and GABA quiet the chatter of wakefulness, allowing neural circuits to replay the patterns of the day, strengthening the connections that matter and pruning those that don't. As the night deepens, levels of norepinephrine and epinephrine drop, giving the brain a rare moment of calm to consolidate memories without the interference of stress signals. Then REM sleep flips the chemical switch: Acetylcholine surges while norepinephrine remains low. This creates a neurochemical landscape ideal for creativity and emotional recalibration. In this state, the mind integrates memories, tests ideas, and reshapes emotions in ways that waking logic never could. The result is a brain that awakens sharper, more inventive, and more emotionally balanced.

Hormones also play a pivotal role in modulating sleep patterns. Unlike neurotransmitters, which are produced in the cell body of a neuron and then transported to its axon (i.e., its proper body), hormones are secreted by various glands in the body and act on various tissues to influence sleep. For example, melatonin is the best-known sleep hormone. The "vampire" hormone as it's known in the sleep community, melatonin is produced by the pineal gland in response to darkness. It signals to the body that it's time to sleep and helps synchronize your circadian rhythm. Melatonin levels rise in the evening and peak during the night, then diminish as morning approaches. It truly acts as a vampire, because it's stifled by sunlight.

Known as the stress hormone, cortisol is released by the adrenal glands and follows a circadian pattern. Its levels are lowest during deep sleep and begin to rise in the early morning, preparing the body for wakefulness. As can be predicted, high cortisol levels at night, often due to stress, can interfere with sleep.

As I mentioned in chapter 1, adenosine is a byproduct of energy consumption in the brain. We can think of it as trash that we dispense in a trashcan. Once it reaches a critical level, it will need to be emptied. Adenosine's levels increase throughout the day as the brain expends energy, creating a sleep pressure or fatigue. This is the basis for the sleep drive: The longer we're awake, the more adenosine builds up, and the threshold for sleep becomes that much stronger. During sleep, adenosine levels decline, allowing the body to feel refreshed upon waking. Then the cycle continues, again and again.

Growth hormone (GH), released during deep sleep, is crucial for tissue repair, muscle growth, and overall recovery. Its secretion is directly linked to slow-wave sleep, emphasizing the importance of this stage of sleep, particularly in children. For example, children with enlarged tonsils and obstructive sleep apnea (OSA) can experience disruptions in growth due to the impact of OSA on GH and overall metabolic function. GH is released in pulses, with the largest secretion occurring during slow-wave sleep. Repeated breathing interruptions, as occur during OSA, disrupt the normal sleep architecture, particularly slow-wave sleep, reducing the time when GH is optimally secreted. Periodic drops in oxygen levels, due to apnea, can impair the hypothalamic-pituitary axis, potentially reducing GH production. OSA also often triggers the release of cortisol, a stress hormone, which can suppress GH secretion and negatively affect growth. In short, then, untreated OSA in children can result in growth retardation due to chronically low levels of growth hormone. Moreover, behavioral and cognitive issues caused by sleep disruption can further affect overall development.

The interaction between neurotransmitters and hormones ensures a seamless transition between sleep stages and the regulation of the sleep-wake cycle. It's like a finely tuned orchestra, conducted by your brain, ensuring the coherence of a beginning, middle, and end. For instance, the reduction of norepinephrine or dopamine (the daytime partygoers) allows GABA and melatonin to dominate, facilitating sleep onset. Conversely, the rise of cortisol in the early morning suppresses melatonin production, signaling to the brain that it's time to wake up.

HOW SLEEP REFINES THE MIND

The night before my biochemistry final as an undergrad I was cramming to learn the entire Krebs cycle like my life depended on it. I stayed up until dawn memorizing every molecule and enzyme, thinking sheer willpower would carry me through. But when I sat down to take the exam, my brain felt foggy, as if someone had scrambled my hippocampus. I couldn't recall half of what I knew earlier. It turns out, I hadn't just pulled an all-nighter—I had also sabotaged the very part of my brain responsible for converting short-term memories into long-term storage. REM sleep is when the brain consolidates complex information; without it, we're basically trying to save files to a hard drive that's unplugged. That was the first time I realized sleep isn't the enemy of achievement; it's the secret weapon. Suffice it to say, that was my last all-nighter. I had learned my lesson all too well and never repeated this lunacy.

If you feel as if your brain is a cluttered desk by the end of the day, that's because your waking hours are filled with new information, conversations, and sensory experiences. During sleep, your brain becomes the ultimate filing clerk, sorting through the day's events, keeping what's important, and discarding the rest.

Memory doesn't just form when we're awake; it solidifies while we sleep. This process happens in two stages. Early in the night, NREM sleep strengthens declarative memory, which includes facts, events, and concepts. If you've ever reviewed flash cards for school or work before bed and found you remembered them better the next day, that's NREM sleep at work.

Later in the night, however, REM sleep dominates and enhances procedural memory, such as how to ride a bike or play a piano piece. It's also essential for integrating information and finding creative solutions to problems. It's as if REM sleep lets our brain connect the dots in ways that we can't while awake. Also, sleep doesn't just help us store memories; it makes them easier to retrieve. Without proper sleep, memories are like files buried deep in a cluttered cabinet. Sleep sharpens the neural pathways that allow us to access more easily what we've learned.

Imagine trying to learn a new language or a complicated dance routine while sleep deprived. Sleep is vital for encoding new information and making it stick. During the day, our brain is flooded with synaptic activity as neurons communicate to absorb new knowledge. By bedtime, our brain is overloaded. Sleep comes to the rescue, as it prunes unnecessary connections and strengthens the essential ones. This process, called synaptic homeostasis, ensures that our brain doesn't max out its capacity.

Even a quick nap can work wonders for learning. A short nap—about twenty to thirty minutes—can sharpen focus and boost learning by giving the brain time to consolidate new information and reset attention. Naps longer than forty-five minutes, however, can push the brain into deeper stages of sleep, leading to grogginess and sluggishness afterward. The sweet spot is the brief "power nap," long enough to refresh the mind but short enough to avoid disrupting the next night's sleep. Sleep is like hitting the "save" button on our mental progress.

If you've ever felt irritable, anxious, or overwhelmed after a poor night's sleep, you've experienced firsthand how sleep impacts emotion regulation. The connection lies in two key areas of the brain: the amygdala and the prefrontal cortex. Think of the amygdala as your brain's alarm system. It detects threats and triggers emotional responses. When you're sleep-deprived, the amygdala becomes hyperactive, overreacting to minor stressors. Have you ever snapped at someone over something trivial after a rough night? I have. We can blame an exhausted amygdala for that response.

Similarly, the prefrontal cortex is like a wise counselor, helping us assess situations rationally and dampen emotional outbursts. Sleep deprivation weakens this region of the brain, leaving us more vulnerable to emotional highs and lows. Together, these effects create a perfect storm: we're more reactive and less able to calm ourselves. One fascinating study used brain imaging to show how sleep affects emotional processing. After a night of poor sleep, participants showed heightened activity in the amygdala and reduced connectivity to the prefrontal cortex. Essentially, the emotional brain hijacked the rational brain.[1]

Even worse, poor sleep interferes with REM sleep, which is when your brain processes and resolves emotional experiences. Without it, negative emotions from the previous day can linger, creating a phenomenon researchers call "emotional carryover."

Sleep isn't just about resting your body. It's about sharpening your mind and balancing your emotions. It consolidates memories, strengthens learning, and keeps our emotional brain in check. It's the quiet powerhouse that makes everything else possible.

THE SLEEP-MOOD CONNECTION

Sleep is often considered a luxury, something to catch up on during the weekend or forgo during busy times. But as you are beginning to understand, sleep is one of the most critical factors in shaping our mental health. Let's explore how sleep, or the lack of it, affects anxiety, depression, and PTSD, three of the most common mental health challenges people face.

Anxiety

Think about the last time you didn't sleep well. Did you feel more on edge, easily irritated, or overwhelmed the next day? I know that I have.

That's no coincidence. Sleep and anxiety are inextricably intertwined and share a complicated relationship that often feels like a vicious cycle. When we don't obtain enough sleep, especially the deep, restorative kind, our brain's ability to regulate emotions diminishes. In fact, it is not stress that usually leads to poor sleep but, rather, poor sleep that lowers our threshold for stress. In fact, a study revealed that although everyone experiences stress when exposed to a stressful event, those who obtained less sleep experienced more stress to low and moderate stressors, whereas the group that obtained adequate sleep did not.[2] The issue here is not about what is stressful or not, but about how a person perceives stress when they don't obtain much sleep. One key player here is the amygdala, the part of your brain responsible for detecting threats. Sleep deprivation causes the amygdala to become hyperactive, making you more sensitive to stressors. Simultaneously, the prefrontal cortex, which helps regulate the amygdala's response, becomes less effective. In other words, we're wired to perceive more danger but less equipped to calm ourselves down.

One study found that sleep-deprived individuals struggled to recognize facial expressions, especially anger and happiness.[3] In other words, when running on empty, your brain has a harder time reading social cues, such as whether someone's annoyed or just mildly irritated. Interestingly, this effect was even stronger in women. The answer to this conundrum lies in neuroscience. The prefrontal cortex is associated with rational thought and reasoning, while the amygdala is all about emotional triggering. With sleep deprivation, the amygdala gains the upper hand and does not allow the prefrontal cortex to balance it out. Think of our brain like a team with a wild, impulsive artist (the amygdala) and a rational, level-headed editor (the prefrontal cortex). When we're well rested, the editor keeps the artist in check, balancing creativity with logic, making sure emotions don't get out of hand. But when we're sleep-deprived, the editor gets sluggish and distracted, letting the artist run wild. Suddenly, everything feels more intense; small frustrations turn into major irritations, and worries feel overwhelming. Without enough sleep, our emotional responses can feel like an unfiltered, messy painting—bold, chaotic, and difficult to control. As this study suggests, sleep deprivation alters the brain's emotional processing, which might explain why everything (and everyone) seems harder to deal with after a rough night of little sleep.

Even one night of poor sleep can increase state anxiety, or temporary feelings of worry. Over time, chronic sleep deprivation can exacerbate trait anxiety, or long-term anxious tendencies. But the silver lining here is that improving sleep, through better habits or targeted therapies, can significantly reduce anxiety. Practices such as breathwork, shadow work, and dreamwork, which I'll elaborate on in part two, not only improve sleep but also reduce anxiety levels.

Depression

If anxiety feels like being stuck in high gear, depression is the opposite: You feel low energy, lack motivation, and have a persistent sense of gloom. Sleep disturbances are almost always part of the equation. It is unclear whether depression propels insomnia or insomnia incites the depression, but whatever the order, it's a vicious cycle that replays itself.

Individuals with depression can experience insomnia, where they struggle to fall or stay asleep, or hypersomnia, where they sleep excessively but still feel fatigued and sleepy. Both conditions disrupt the natural rhythm of the body, especially the circadian system.

Sleep doesn't just rest the body: It restores emotional balance at the molecular level. In the quiet hours of the night, serotonin and dopamine are replenished and retuned, like instruments in an orchestra preparing for the next day's performance. When sleep is scarce, their harmonies falter: Serotonin loses its steadiness, dopamine its spark. The world looks dimmer; joy feels distant. But as sleep deepens and returns, those inner instruments find their pitch again, and the mind remembers what it feels like to be in tune with itself.

Interestingly, some treatments for depression, such as sleep deprivation therapy, involve restricting sleep temporarily. Why? Because for some people, a night of sleep deprivation can trigger a rapid, albeit temporary, improvement in mood. Researchers believe this might reset certain brain circuits, though the effect isn't fully understood.

Post-Traumatic Stress Disorder

For individuals with post-traumatic stress disorder (PTSD), sleep, ironically, can be both a refuge and a battlefield. Nightmares are a hallmark symptom of PTSD, replaying traumatic events in vivid, often terrifying detail. As expected, these nightmares disrupt REM sleep, the stage associated with emotional processing and memory consolidation.

Here's the catch, though: REM sleep is essential for "filing away" traumatic memories in a way that reduces their emotional intensity. Without proper REM sleep, these memories remain raw and intrusive, perpetuating the symptoms of PTSD. Furthermore, individuals with PTSD often develop a hypervigilant sleep pattern, never fully relaxing into slow-wave sleep because their brains are on high alert. This makes them more likely to wake frequently during the night, further reducing the restorative power of sleep.

One fascinating area of research involves using therapies such as eye movement desensitization and reprocessing (EMDR), dream rehearsal therapy, or even medications to reduce nightmares. Dream rehearsal therapy is especially fascinating. It's one of the most practical and surprisingly simple ways to reshape nightmares. The idea is to rewrite the dream while you're awake—changing its script, setting, or ending—and then mentally rehearse the new version before sleep. For example, someone who keeps dreaming they're being chased might imagine turning around, facing the pursuer, or stepping into a safe place instead. Over time, the brain learns to replace the old fear memory with the new narrative, and the nightmare loses its grip. It's a reminder that even in sleep, the mind is trainable—that we can participate in our own healing stories.

What ties all this together is the role sleep plays in emotional regulation. Sleep isn't just about physical recovery; it's when our brain processes emotions, resolves conflicts, and resets itself. During REM sleep, for example, the brain activates the default mode network that helps integrate emotional memories into our broader sense of self. When sleep is disrupted, our brain loses its ability to do this emotional housekeeping. Over time, this leads to heightened emotional reactivity, poor decision-making, and an increased risk of mental health challenges.

It's tempting to think of sleep as a passive state, something our body does when we're not awake. But sleep is an active, dynamic process that deeply influences our mental health. For anxiety, sleep helps our brain recalibrate its threat detection system. For depression, it restores the balance of mood-regulating transmitters. And for PTSD, it's essential for processing trauma and reducing emotional pain.

If you're struggling with anxiety, depression, or PTSD, improving your sleep could be one of the most consequential steps you take. It might not solve all your problems, but it lays a solid foundation for healing and resilience. So tonight, when you're tempted to stay up late scrolling through your phone, remember that sleep isn't just good for your body; it's also essential for your mind.

3

COMMON SLEEP DISORDERS

INSOMNIA

MY FIRST TRUE BOUT OF INSOMNIA AS AN ADULT OCCURRED on a specific night that I still recall. That night, sleep didn't just slip away. It bolted, tore itself from me like flesh from bone. I lay there, rigid and hot, with my mind cracking open to things I hadn't thought about in years. My grandfather's face surfaced—his comforting smell, his large teeth, the way he would cup my face in his calloused hands and call me *azizam* ("my dear"). He had been my whole world when I was a kid in Iran, before the noise, before we left everything behind during the Islamic Revolution. I remembered the exact way his voice dropped when he said goodbye at the airport, how I didn't understand it was forever. He died shortly after I completed my sleep medicine fellowship, and I never told anyone how much that gutted me. A week after his death, insomnia hit me. I stared at the ceiling like it might open and swallow me. Every time I closed my eyes, his face returned. I didn't want to sleep; I wanted to go back. But you can't go back. You just lie there. Awake. Waiting.

Insomnia is the most common sleep disorder, and many of us will experience it either acutely or chronically in our lifetime. It is characterized by difficulty initiating, maintaining, or obtaining restorative sleep, despite adequate opportunities. Insomnia often gets confused with sleep deprivation, but sleep deprivation usually means you can't sleep because you're not giving yourself enough time (perhaps because you stayed up binge-watching a show or working late), while insomnia means you're trying to sleep and just can't, even when you have the chance. It's a frustrating disconnect between the body and the brain. It's not about laziness or bad habits; it's about a hyperalert mind that just won't shut off, even when you're exhausted.

Insomnia can leave you wrestling with consequences in your waking life, including fatigue, irritability, poor concentration, and even anxiety, depression, and cognitive impairment. For many, insomnia can be acute, lasting days to weeks, often due to stress or temporary disruptions. On the other hand, up to 30 percent of the population experiences chronic insomnia, which occurs at least three times a week for three months or longer.

So, what's behind this relentless wakefulness? Insomnia can be triggered by a tangled web of psychological, physiological, and environmental factors, each playing its own role in keeping us awake. Let's take a look at some of them.

Rumination and Cortisol Spikes

One of the most common reasons people can't fall asleep—including my patients—isn't anything physical; it's that their brain just won't shut off. Ruminating thoughts are like a late-night talk show that no one asked for, but it airs anyway. You lie down, ready to drift off, and suddenly your mind opens a tab for every unresolved situation you've experienced in the past several years. Or it replays tomorrow's to-do list like a broken record, with increasingly unrealistic demands and imagined disasters. This kind of mental looping isn't just annoying; it's a hallmark of what keeps so many people up at night.

These ruminations often feel urgent, like problems that must be solved *right now*. The truth is that the brain isn't designed to solve things effectively when it's supposed to be sleeping. Instead, it gets stuck, chewing the same thought over and over, making sleep feel impossible. Sometimes it generates low-grade anxiety. Sometimes it stirs up guilt. Sometimes it just treats the quiet of bedtime as the perfect moment to overanalyze your entire existence and what it means. Our brains are wired for such contemplations, but not when it's time to sleep. The irony is, the more we try to force sleep to come, the louder those thoughts seem to get. As we start to fall asleep, our brain shifts from using the prefrontal cortex—the area responsible for logic and decision-making—to more limbic and default mode networks, which are tied to emotion and free association. Keeping your prefrontal cortex engaged creates a vicious cycle that leaves you staring at the ceiling or the clock night after night.

We may also ruminate about others, imagining their lives as richer, easier, or more fulfilled than our own. "Look at those Instagram pics! Look at how great their life is!" you think. "I'm missing out on that glamour." Alone in the dark, we forget that everyone's life is uncomfortable in some way; it may not resemble our own discomfort, but it's there. As we know, no period of comfort will last. Everything is fleeting, everything is short-lived, even discomfort. Looking at the situation this way, reminding ourselves that things are not necessarily as they appear, helps us recognize that our rumination is futile.

Women struggle with insomnia more than men. Research has found that women are more likely to engage in rumination, a pattern of repetitive, often negative thinking, which can keep the mind overly active at night and make it harder to sleep. In fact, the anterior and posterior cingulate cortex were activated longer in women after an experiment in which they were prompted to work faster in their performance during an arithmetic task.[1] While men might distract themselves from stress, women are more likely to internalize it, especially when anxious. This mental loop, combined with hormonal fluctuations, could help explain why sleep struggles hit women harder and more often.

Rumination can also cause the release of cortisol, a metabolic hormone that signals to the body that it needs glucose. When the body signals to the brain that there's an emergency (sending you into fight, flight, or freeze mode), cortisol acts to mobilize more energy, more glucose for you to use to face the stressor. Although this can be beneficial, if you are chronically stressed, you will continue to secrete more cortisol, and your body will constantly be in an activated state, making falling and staying asleep more difficult. If your thoughts and fears about the past and future keep swirling, they keep generating cortisol, and insomnia ensues. You're left there, in bed, not only thinking about the problem that you have been attempting to solve (even though it is ultimately unsolvable in that moment) but also ruminating about not being able to sleep. In essence, you create two problems out of an unsolvable one, doubling your anxiety and worsening your insomnia. You're left believing that you just can't win, that you're cursed with your insomnia, and the cycle continues.

Sleep Reactivity

Sleep reactivity, which is how sensitive our sleep is to stress, is another concept that may explain why certain individuals develop chronic insomnia while others don't. Some people, when they're under pressure or dealing with emotional turmoil, can still crash and sleep through the night. Others—those with high sleep reactivity—find that even mild stressors flip a switch, making it difficult to fall or stay asleep. This trait is a big predictor of who might develop insomnia, especially chronic insomnia. From an evolutionary standpoint, sleep reactivity may have been a useful survival mechanism. If our brain stayed on high alert during times of danger, like when predators were nearby or the tribe was under threat, staying awake could have kept us alive. But in the modern world, where the threats are more psychological than physical, this hair-trigger arousal system backfires, keeping individuals awake over a work deadline or a breakup. In a way, then, insomnia might be the shadow of an ancient vigilance system that once served us well but no longer does.

Paradoxical Insomnia

In the sleep clinic, among the true insomniacs, I also see patients who swear they haven't slept a wink all night, but when we do a sleep study, it turns out they slept a decent amount. This is what we call paradoxical insomnia. It's not that they're making it up; their brains genuinely *feel* awake, even when their bodies are asleep. It's a fascinating disconnect that reminds me how complex and subjective sleep really is. Most of the time, when these individuals are confronted with the objective data that their sleep is normal, or not as bad as they thought, their insomnia improves, often significantly.

Individuals with insomnia have a chronic sleep debt. But as I mentioned in chapter 1, this debt cannot be made up by simply sleeping more on the weekends. Sleep doesn't work like a savings account that you can deposit money into and then withdraw whenever necessary. You can't save up on sleep because sleep, as you have seen, works on a different dynamic. It'll give to you freely, if you just let it.

Biological Misfires

In chapter 2, we discussed the importance of the two-process model of sleep regulation where process S (homeostatic sleep drive) and process C (circadian rhythm) work independently but in a beautifully choreographed dance to regulate wakefulness and sleep. When these processes are not working properly, insomnia can be the result.

In process S, the drive to sleep gradually builds during the day as adenosine and other neurochemicals accumulate in the brain. It's as if your body is making a natural anesthetic that will induce you to sleep once it reaches a certain threshold. Poor sleep hygiene or naps can reduce this sleep pressure or drive, making it more difficult to fall asleep at bedtime. Also, hyperarousal, which commonly accompanies insomnia, can override the natural homeostatic drive, delaying sleep or leading to fragmented sleep.

In process C, the body's internal clock is governed by the suprachiasmatic nucleus (SCN) and regulates alertness and sleepiness over a twenty-four-hour cycle. It is influenced by light exposure and melatonin secretion. When this inner clock drifts out of tune with the world around you, even the simple act of falling asleep can feel like swimming against the current.

Process S and process C are two distinct processes, but their interplay determines whether you're sleepy or awake. For example, if you wake up refreshed in the morning, having had restorative sleep, you've depleted your adenosine level and so your process S begins anew: Your sleep drive is at its lowest because your brain has cleared the accumulated adenosine. At that point, your process C is also at a high level, suggesting maximal alertness. At the other end of the day, when you're preparing to sleep, your adenosine level has had a chance to build up and is at its highest level, while your circadian rhythm is at its lowest, making sleep that much easier.

When the two processes function as they should, you get a seamless sleep. However, in individuals with insomnia, irregular sleep patterns can weaken process S, compounding the problem. In a similar pattern, one that I often see in clinical practice, stress and anxiety can disrupt both processes by suppressing the natural decline of alertness (process C) and reducing the ability to build or sustain sleep pressure (process S).

You may wonder why process S wouldn't just continue to build, making you more and more sleepy instead of sleepless. It does, but because the two processes work independently from each other, process C pays no attention to how sleepy you feel. If your circadian rhythm is out of sync or misaligned with your level of sleepiness, they're like two ships passing in the night, and you get to be awake to see it.

Revenge Bedtime Procrastination

In our modern age, those of us who are overtaxed with work during the day may use our nights to regain some of that free time back. It's understandable that when we have so much to do, something must give; time must be found elsewhere. *Revenge bedtime procrastination* is a relatively new term that describes staying up late to reclaim time for yourself—for reading, hobbies, binge-watching, going out with friends, paying bills, and so on—things your daytime obligations prevent you from doing. As you can imagine, such "revenge on time" can be counterproductive because you interfere with your circadian rhythm. Many of these activities leave you feeling wired and unable to wind down. Trying to regain this time back at night will, ironically, make you lose time and productivity the following day, and possibly cause chronic insomnia. What would be infinitely more productive is to create short breaks throughout the day so that you can accomplish things before the evening, when winding down should be a priority.

TREATMENTS FOR INSOMNIA

Cognitive behavioral therapy for insomnia (CBT-I) is considered the gold-standard treatment for chronic insomnia. I've used it successfully with many patients and even wrote a book about it called *Sleep Reimagined*. However, it doesn't work for everyone. Many cannot adhere to its regimented schedule or, for reasons we don't quite understand, they just don't get results. If this treatment hasn't worked for you, or you want to try something different, there are several non-traditional therapies for insomnia that are backed by science. Let's dive into a few options that might surprise you.

Herbal Remedies for Insomnia

If you've struggled with insomnia and been to a sleep doctor, they probably prescribed you a medication such as benzodiazepines (lorazepam and diazepam) and benzodiazepine receptor agonists (zolpidem, zaleplon, eszopiclone—the so-called Z-drugs, because the letter *z* appears in their generic names). These all have untoward side effects, including feeling groggy the next day. They also carry a small risk of parasomnias, such as eating or even driving without remembering it (I'll cover parasomnias later in this chapter). Furthermore, there is a risk of tolerance—the necessity of increasing dosage (and overmedicating) to maintain the same effect—and rebound insomnia in which sudden discontinuation of the agent can cause a worsening of the original symptoms.[2] In lieu of these agents, we should ask whether nature can help you rest. The idea of turning to herbal remedies for insomnia has been around for centuries, and in today's well-focused world, it's no surprise that these ancient practices are getting a modern spotlight. From calming teas to capsules promising sweet dreams, the question remains: Do they work? Let's take a look.

VALERIAN ROOT

Valerian root (*Valeriana officinalis*) has been used since the time of ancient Greece to treat insomnia and anxiety. Derived from the root of the valerian plant, it's often consumed as a tea, tincture, or supplement. It's thought to increase gamma-aminobutyric acid (GABA) levels in the brain. GABA is a neurotransmitter that calms the nervous system—the brake, if you will—helping your brain transition into a relaxed state ideal for sleep. A meta-analysis found that valerian root improved sleep quality compared to placebo in people with mild insomnia.[3] However, not all studies are glowing. Some research suggests that effects may be modest and take a few weeks of consistent use to notice. You can try it by drinking valerian tea thirty minutes to an hour before bed or taking it as a supplement (usually 300 to 600 mg). Start with a low dose to avoid side effects such as dizziness or drowsiness the next day.

CHAMOMILE AND APIGENIN

Chamomile tea is the ultimate bedtime classic. Known for its gentle, calming properties, chamomile is derived from the dried flowers of the *Matricaria chamomilla* plant. It contains an antioxidant called apigenin that binds to certain receptors in your brain to promote relaxation and reduce anxiety. A 2017 study showed that elderly participants who drank chamomile tea had improved sleep quality compared to those who didn't.[4] You can start by brewing a cup of chamomile tea and sipping it an hour before bed. For stronger effects, you can try concentrated chamomile supplements.

If you've ever sipped chamomile tea before bed, you're already familiar with apigenin, even if you didn't realize it. Apigenin is a flavonoid found in chamomile that binds to GABA receptors in the brain, essentially dialing down overactive neurons and encouraging relaxation. What's great about apigenin is that it's not just for sleep; it also has anti-inflammatory and antioxidant properties, so it's also beneficial for your overall health. However, don't expect apigenin to knock you out like a sleeping pill. Apigenin's effects are gentle, making it an excellent option if you're dealing with mild stress or occasional sleeplessness. You can get apigenin from chamomile tea, but for a stronger punch, some supplements offer concentrated doses.

PASSIONFLOWER

Passionflower (*Passiflora incarnata*) is a climbing vine known for its stunning purple flowers and its ability to calm an overactive mind. Like valerian, passionflower increases GABA levels in the brain, reducing restlessness and anxiety. It's particularly helpful for people whose insomnia stems from rumination. A 2011 study found that people who drank passionflower tea for a week reported better sleep quality than those who drank a placebo tea.[5] Passionflower is available as a tea, tincture, or capsule. A soothing cup of passionflower tea before bed might just quiet your mind enough to drift off.

LAVENDER

Lavender, which is often associated with spa treatments, has a long history of being used to promote relaxation and improve sleep. Its calming effects are linked to compounds such as linalool, which interacts with the brain to reduce stress and encourage sleep. One study found that lavender oil improved sleep quality and reduced fatigue in participants with insomnia.[6] You can try lavender in several ways. Diffuse lavender essential oil in your bedroom or add a few drops of it to your pillow or bedtime bath. Some teas and supplements also include lavender for its calming effects.

ASHWAGANDHA

Ashwagandha (*Withania somnifera*) is known as the stress buster. It's an adaptogenic herb that helps the body cope with stress. It has been used in Ayurvedic medicine for centuries to promote relaxation and better sleep. The active compound in ashwagandha, triethylene glycol, has sedative effects that may improve sleep quality and duration. A 2021 study found that people who took ashwagandha extract experienced significant improvements in sleep quality and felt more refreshed in the morning, likely because ashwagandha reduces cortisol levels (the stress hormone), making it easier to wind down at night.[7] This herb is typically taken as a capsule or powder. The recommended dose for sleep support is around 300 to 600 mg of standardized extract per day.

LEMON BALM

Lemon balm is a member of the mint family, with a mild lemon scent that's as soothing as its effects on the body. It, too, increases GABA activity in the brain, promoting a sense of calm and reducing insomnia linked to anxiety. One study found that lemon balm extract, also known as *Melissa officinalis*, reduced symptoms of anxiety and improved sleep after fifteen days of use.[8] Lemon balm can be taken as a tea, tincture, or supplement. It's often combined with other calming herbs such as valerian or chamomile for a synergistic effect.

GREEN TEA

If you've ever wondered why green tea feels soothing despite its caffeine content, look to L-theanine, an amino acid that promotes relaxation without sedation. It works by boosting alpha brain waves, which are associated with a calm, focused state of mind, and increasing levels of calming neurotransmitters such as GABA, serotonin, and dopamine. L-theanine is particularly useful if your insomnia stems from a racing mind. It helps you wind down without feeling groggy the next morning, making it a fantastic choice for people who need mental clarity during the day. You can even combine it with magnesium or melatonin for an even more potent sleep-supporting effect.

HOPS

Hops (*Humulus lupulus*) are best known as a key ingredient in beer, but they've been used for centuries as a natural sedative. The flowers of the hop plant contain compounds such as humulone and lupulone, which have mild sedative and anxiolytic effects. Hops are often paired with valerian root in sleep supplements because they seem to enhance each other's effects. If you've ever had an herbal tea or tincture with both, you might have noticed a soothing warmth that eases you into sleep. For those who prefer avoiding alcohol, this is a great way to get the calming benefits of hops without the beer buzz.

MAGNOLIA BARK

Magnolia bark has been used in Traditional Chinese Medicine for centuries to address anxiety and sleep issues. It contains compounds such as honokiol and magnolol, which can reduce cortisol levels and encourage relaxation. What's unique about magnolia bark is its ability to help with nocturnal awakenings. If you're someone who falls asleep easily but can't stay asleep, this might be a good option for you.

UNUSUAL SUPPLEMENTS

Not exactly an herb, but worth mentioning, glycine is an amino acid that helps lower core body temperature, a crucial signal for sleep. It also supports the production of serotonin, which is converted into melatonin. Studies show that taking glycine before bed can improve sleep quality and help us feel more refreshed in the morning.[9]

Agar 35 and Vimala (also known as Bimala) are herbal formulations used in Tibetan sleep medicine to promote relaxation and support a better night's sleep. Agar 35 typically features extracts from agarwood, an ingredient prized in traditional medicine for its calming, sedative properties, combined with other natural botanicals. Vimala, on the other hand, is an Ayurvedic blend that often includes herbs such as ashwagandha, Brahmi (*Bacopa monnieri*), and Jatamansi (*Nardostachys jatamansi*), all known for their ability to reduce anxiety and enhance mental calmness. These supplements can be used to wean you off your traditional hypnotics, creating less rebound insomnia.[10]

Nontraditional Treatments for Insomnia

ACUPUNCTURE

Acupuncture, rooted in Traditional Chinese Medicine, involves inserting fine needles into specific points on the body to restore balance and promote healing. It can regulate the body's stress response, improve blood flow, and increase production of sleep-promoting hormones such as melatonin. It's also thought to calm the nervous system, which can be overactive in people with insomnia. A 2025 meta-analysis found that acupuncture significantly improved sleep quality and reduced insomnia severity compared to sham acupuncture.[11] Studies suggest that it's particularly effective for people with chronic insomnia or stress-related sleep issues. Work with a licensed acupuncturist who has experience treating sleep disorders. You may notice improvement after just a few sessions, though consistency is key.

BRIGHT LIGHT THERAPY

Bright light therapy can be useful for resetting your inner clock. This type of therapy isn't just for seasonal affective disorder; it can also help regulate your sleep-wake cycle. Our circadian rhythm, or internal clock, relies on light cues to regulate sleep. Misalignment of this rhythm can cause insomnia, and bright light therapy can help reset it. For example, if you're struggling with delayed sleep phase (falling asleep too late), exposure to bright light in the morning can help you feel sleepy earlier at night. Light therapy can effectively improve sleep onset, duration, and overall quality, especially for insomnia related to circadian rhythm disorders. Use a light therapy box that emits 10,000 lux of white or blue light. Sit near the box for twenty to thirty minutes in the morning to reap the benefits.

ESSENTIAL OILS

Essential oils, particularly those known for their calming properties, can promote relaxation and better sleep. Scents such as lavender and chamomile are thought to activate calming pathways in the brain and reduce anxiety, a common contributor to insomnia. Aromatherapy combined with relaxation techniques has been shown to enhance its effects. Use a diffuser in your bedroom to disperse calming essential oils before bed. Alternatively, apply diluted lavender oil to your pulse points or pillow.

MINDFULNESS AND MEDITATION

While mindfulness and meditation might seem mainstream these days, they're still underutilized as tools for insomnia. Mindfulness helps because it focuses on bringing attention to the present moment, reducing racing thoughts and worries that keep us awake. Practices such as guided meditations or body scans help calm your nervous system and prepare our body for sleep. A 2015 study found that mindfulness-based interventions significantly improved sleep quality and reduced symptoms of insomnia compared to standard sleep education. Participants also reported reduced stress and improved daytime functioning.[12] You can find many sleep-focused meditations online or on apps such as Calm, Insight Timer, or Headspace. You can also try a simple self-guided body scan when you get into bed: Focus on relaxing each part of your body, starting from your toes and working upward.

WEIGHTED BLANKETS

Weighted blankets have gained popularity for their calming effects, and there's some science to bolster their claims. The gentle pressure of a weighted blanket mimics a therapeutic technique called deep pressure stimulation, which can reduce anxiety and promote relaxation. This can lead to a calmer state, making it easier to fall and stay asleep.

A 2020 study found that weighted blankets improved sleep quality in people with insomnia and reduced symptoms of anxiety.[13] Choose a blanket that's about 10 percent of your body weight. Use it during the night or while winding down before bed.

HYPNOTHERAPY

Hypnotherapy for insomnia involves guided relaxation and suggestions to reframe negative thought patterns about sleep. It can lower stress, reduce arousal, and help train our mind to associate bed with relaxation rather than frustration. A 2014 study found that hypnotherapy significantly improved deep sleep duration in participants, which is crucial for feeling rested.[14] Hypnosis can also address underlying anxiety or trauma that contributes to insomnia. If you want to try this method, look for a licensed hypnotherapist or use apps that provide sleep-focused hypnosis sessions.

TAI CHI AND QIGONG

Tai chi and qigong are ancient practices that combine slow, deliberate movements with focused breathing, offering both physical and mental relaxation. Regular practice reduces stress, calms the nervous system, and improves overall sleep quality. They're especially helpful for older adults or those with chronic conditions contributing to insomnia. A 2016 review concluded that tai chi improves sleep quality and reduces symptoms of insomnia, particularly in older adults.[15] Join a local class or follow online tutorials designed for beginners. Even ten to fifteen minutes a day can make a significant difference in how you sleep.

Insomnia can be exhausting to treat, but the world of nontraditional therapies offers hope. From acupuncture needles to the gentle weight of a blanket, these approaches provide scientifically proven options that cater to different needs and preferences. If one of these resonates with you, give it a try. Don't be afraid to explore the path less traveled.

WHEN SLEEP TAKES YOUR BREATH AWAY

Sleep-disordered breathing (SDB) refers to conditions in which airflow is disrupted during sleep, with obstructive sleep apnea (OSA) being the most common.[16] If you've ever heard someone snore loudly, gasp, or even stop breathing for brief moments in their sleep, you've witnessed what sleep apnea can look and sound like. But why does this happen, and why does it matter?

At its core, OSA occurs when the airway becomes partially or completely blocked during sleep. The mechanics of this process are surprisingly simple. During sleep, especially in REM stages, the muscles in your throat and tongue relax. In some individuals, this relaxation goes too far, causing the soft tissues to collapse and obstruct airflow. When this happens, the brain senses a drop in oxygen levels and briefly wakes you up, sometimes just for a second, to reopen the airway. These interruptions, called apneas (complete blockage) or hypopneas (partial blockage), can happen dozens or even hundreds of times per night in severe cases. The result: The sleeper is often unaware of these arousals, but their sleep becomes fragmented and unrefreshing.

More than just an annoyance or a snoring issue, SDB can wreak havoc on the body and mind and can cause significant cardiovascular strain. Each cycle of apnea, hypopnea, and arousal triggers a fight-or-flight response, releasing stress hormones such as adrenaline. Over time, this repeated stress increases the risk of hypertension, heart disease, and stroke, to name a few. Fragmented sleep also means less time spent in the deep, restorative stages of sleep, including slow-wave and REM sleep. This leads to excessive daytime sleepiness, reduced concentration, and slower reaction times. Furthermore, interrupted sleep can disrupt hormone balance, making it more difficult to regulate hunger and glucose levels, increasing the risk of obesity and type 2 diabetes. Poor sleep also impairs memory, learning, and emotional regulation. Many individuals with untreated SDB report irritability, anxiety, and even depression. In children, OSA presents with symptoms like attention deficit hyperactivity disorder (ADHD). Clinicians should consider pediatric OSA whenever a child shows signs of irritability or poor attention.

Interestingly, women often present with sleep apnea in a more subtle and less classic way than men. Instead of loud snoring and obvious gasping, they're more likely to report insomnia, fatigue, morning headaches, or mood changes such as anxiety or depression. Hormonal differences, smaller airway structures, and how fat is distributed around the neck and upper body all play a role in how sleep apnea shows up—and gets missed—in women. When I evaluate women with insomnia in my sleep clinic, I always consider the possibility that sleep apnea could be the culprit of those fragmented and restless nights.

While we've come a long way in understanding the physiology of and consequences of SDB, there are still many unanswered questions. For example, why do some individuals with severe sleep apnea have minimal symptoms, while others with mild apnea feel profoundly impacted? Is SDB causing conditions such as hypertension, or do these conditions exacerbate SDB? The relationship isn't always clear.

Our understanding of sleep-disordered breathing is a modern development, but cultures throughout history have noted phenomena that might be describing SDB. The Greeks and Romans recognized "sleep suffocation" and "snoring-related disturbances" in some writings, although these were often attributed to an imbalance of humors or spiritual forces.[17] In medieval Europe, descriptions of "night hags" sitting on a sleeper's chest might align with the gasping and choking sensations associated with apnea, although they were interpreted as supernatural attacks.[18]

It wasn't until the twentieth century that sleep medicine emerged as a distinct field, with technologies such as polysomnography, or sleep studies, making it possible to objectively study sleep and its disorders.

Today, we recognize sleep apnea as a common condition affecting millions worldwide, but historical and cultural interpretations remind us that our understanding of health is always evolving and in flux.

The gold-standard treatment for SDB is positive airway pressure (PAP) therapy, such as CPAP, BiPAP, or adaptive servo-ventilation (ASV). Other treatment options include devices that you place in your mouth, such as a mandibular advancement device (MAD), which propels the jaw forward to create more space in the back of the throat. Recently, a medication (tirzepatide, or Zepbound) was approved by the US Food and Drug Administration (FDA) for the treatment of moderate to severe OSA in adults with obesity, to be used in combination with a reduced-calorie diet and increased physical activity. Tirzapetide works by activating receptors of hormones secreted from the intestine (glucagon-like peptide-1 or GLP-1) and glucose-dependent insulinotropic polypeptide (GIP) to reduce appetite and food intake. By reducing body weight, studies show that Zepbound also improves OSA.

Sleep position also matters. For most people, sleeping on their side, especially the left side, tends to offer the most benefits. It can improve digestion, reduce snoring, and lower the risk of heartburn. It also helps keep the airway more open compared to sleeping on your back. Back sleeping might work well for spinal alignment but can worsen snoring and cause sleep-disordered breathing. Stomach sleeping is generally the least recommended because it can strain your neck and lower back.

Alternative Treatments for Sleep-Disordered Breathing

In addition to medical interventions, there are also alternative, evidence-based treatments for SDB that provide hope for those looking for something beyond traditional methods.

DIGERIDOO

The didgeridoo, a traditional wind instrument of the Aboriginal people of Australia, has gained scientific recognition as a potential therapy for OSA. Playing the didgeridoo involves circular breathing, a technique that strengthens the muscles in our upper airway and throat. Since weak or collapsed throat muscles are a major cause of OSA, toning them can reduce apneas and improve sleep. A 2006 study found that participants who played the didgeridoo regularly experienced fewer apneas and less daytime sleepiness compared to a control group.[19] Researchers attributed the improvement to better airway muscle tone and reduced airway collapse. Today, you can easily access lessons and tutorials online.

SINGING

Like the digeridoo, singing can also help tone the muscles in your throat and soft palate. Certain vocal exercises strengthen and coordinate the muscles that keep your airway open during sleep. Singing is particularly useful for mild to moderate OSA or snoring. A robust study found that singing exercises improved snoring, mild to moderate sleep apnea, and sleepiness over a three-month period by strengthening pharyngeal musculature, or the airway muscles.[20] Focus on exercises that involve sustained vowel sounds or specific tones. Singing in the shower counts!

MYOFUNCTIONAL THERAPY

Myofunctional therapy, also known as orofacial exercises, involves targeted movements to strengthen the tongue, cheeks, and throat—such as pressing your tongue against the roof of your mouth or repeating certain tongue movements. These exercises help reposition the tongue and improve muscle tone in the upper airway, making it less likely to collapse during sleep. This type of therapy is particularly effective for people with mild OSA or those who can't tolerate PAP therapy. Think of it as yoga for your mouth. A 2015 meta-analysis showed that myofunctional therapy significantly reduced the severity of OSA and snoring.[21] You can work with a trained therapist or find guided exercises online.

PRANAYAMA

Breathing techniques such as the yogic practice of *pranayama* can also improve SDB. Focused nasal breathing helps strengthen the diaphragm and improve airflow, especially in people with nasal obstructions or who habitually breathe through their mouths. Practices such as alternate nostril breathing promote relaxation, which can improve sleep quality overall. While large-scale studies are limited, small trials suggest that pranayama can reduce SDB and improve oxygen levels in individuals with mild OSA. Start with a simple breathing practice: Inhale deeply through one nostril while closing the other with your finger, then switch sides. Practicing on your own can be grounding and restorative, but approach it gently; breathwork can sometimes shift your state of consciousness more than you expect, especially if you're new to it.

ACUPUNCTURE

A cornerstone of Traditional Chinese Medicine, acupuncture has shown promise in alleviating OSA symptoms in some studies. It is believed to stimulate nerves and muscles in the throat, improving tone and reducing airway obstruction. It may also help regulate breathing patterns and improve sleep quality. A recent review and meta-analysis found that acupuncture can improve OSA.[22] If you're contemplating this option, work with a licensed acupuncturist who has experience treating sleep disorders.

POSITIONAL THERAPY

If your SDB is worse when you sleep on your back (this is called positional OSA), changing your sleep position can be a game changer. Sleeping on your side prevents your tongue and soft tissues from collapsing into the airway. Use a wedge pillow or body pillow to help you maintain your position throughout the night. Special devices, such as wearable position trainers, vibrate gently to remind you to roll back to your side if you roll onto your back. Studies have shown that positional therapy can significantly reduce OSA symptoms in positional cases.

Treating OSA isn't a one-size-fits-all answer. While PAP and traditional therapies remain gold standards, these alternative treatments offer exciting, scientifically supported options if you are seeking something different or looking to supplement your current treatment. From playing a didgeridoo to nasal breathing exercises, these methods can empower you to take control of your sleep health while honoring practices rooted in cultural and creative traditions.

If you're curious about trying any of these options, consult your doctor or sleep specialist to see what a good fit for your needs might be. You might discover that the road to better sleep and breathing leads through music, movement, or mindfulness.

PARASOMNIAS

Imagine waking up in the middle of the night to find someone cooking an elaborate meal, yelling in terror, or calmly walking around the house—all while they're still fast asleep. These behaviors belong to a fascinating category of sleep disorders known as parasomnias. Parasomnias are strange and sometimes dramatic activities that occur during sleep and provide a window into the complexity of the sleeping brain. Let's unpack what they are, why they occur, and how different cultures have interpreted them over time.

Parasomnias are involuntary physical or verbal behaviors that arise during sleep or the transitions between sleep and wakefulness. They are categorized based on the stage of sleep during which they occur. For example, sleepwalking (somnambulism), sleep terrors, and confusional arousals occur during the deeper stages of NREM sleep, typically in the first half of the night, and are more common in children, presumably because of the greater amount of slow-wave sleep in that population. On the other hand, REM parasomnias, which include REM sleep behavior disorder (RBD) and nightmares, arise during REM sleep, the stage when dreaming is most vivid. Other parasomnias—for example, sleep-related eating disorder—can occur at any point during the night.

The exact causes of parasomnias aren't fully understood, but they appear to involve a partial arousal of the brain. During these episodes, parts of the brain responsible for motor activity and emotional processing may "wake up" while the areas controlling conscious thought remain asleep.

With sleepwalking, which occurs during deep NREM sleep, the person may walk, perform tasks, or even leave the house, but they typically won't recall the event. Sleep terrors are intense episodes of fear, screaming, and physical agitations, which also occur during NREM sleep. Unlike nightmares, the individual doesn't awaken fully or recall the terror afterward. In REM sleep, most people experience temporary paralysis to prevent acting out dreams. In RBD, this paralysis is incomplete, allowing people to physically enact their dreams, which can occasionally result in injury. This diagnosis can predate a neurodegenerative disorder such as Parkinson's disease by approximately a decade. Risk factors for parasomnias include genetics, sleep deprivation, stress, and use of alcohol. Conditions such as sleep apnea or restless legs syndrome can also increase their likelihood.

Throughout history, parasomnias have been viewed through a variety of lenses, from the mystical to the medical. In ancient Greece and Rome, sleepwalking was sometimes seen as evidence of divine intervention or a connection to the spiritual realm. Sleep terrors and other disturbing nocturnal behaviors were often attributed to demonic possession or curses in many cultures, including medieval Europe. Scandinavian tales described the *mara,* a supernatural being that sat on sleepers' chests, causing terrifying dreams or sleep paralysis. Most famously, sleepwalking was referenced in literature, as in Shakespeare's *Macbeth,* where Lady Macbeth's somnambulism reflects her guilt and inner turmoil. Today, parasomnias are understood as neurological phenomena, though cultural interpretations persist. For example, in some parts of the world, sleepwalking may still be seen as a sign of spiritual unrest or an omen.

Parasomnias are a testament to how dynamic and unpredictable sleep can be. Whether it's a child crying out in a sleep terror, an adult dreaming so vividly they act it out, or the sleepwalker navigating their environment with eerie precision, these episodes remind us that sleep is far from passive. Kenneth Parks's case is one of the most chilling and fascinating examples of sleepwalking gone horribly wrong. Back in 1987, this Toronto man drove fourteen miles in a sleepwalking state, entered his in-laws' home, and tragically killed his mother-in-law while injuring his father-in-law. The wild part? Parks had no memory of it. What makes this even more startling is that the court ultimately found him not guilty due to automatism; basically, he wasn't conscious of his actions, so he couldn't be criminally responsible. It's one of those real-life cases that blurs the line between medicine, morality, and law; and it still sparks debates about sleep disorders and criminal responsibility today.

Conventional treatments for parasomnias consist of both behavioral and environmental adjustments. A consistent sleep routine reduces the risk of parasomnias by stabilizing one's sleep cycles. Stress is also a common trigger for night terrors and sleepwalking, so techniques including deep breathing, yoga, or therapy can help. For sleepwalkers, securing the environment by locking doors, clearing tripping hazards, and installing alarms is helpful in preventing injuries.

Medication isn't always necessary, but in severe cases, it can be a useful tool. Benzodiazepines, such as clonazepam, are commonly used for REM sleep behavior disorder (RBD) or severe night terrors, as they can calm the brain and reduce episodes. For parasomnias linked to anxiety or depression, certain antidepressants can help regulate sleep. Melatonin, the sleep hormone, may also improve RBD by stabilizing REM cycles. Cognitive behavioral therapy can be effective for addressing the triggers behind parasomnias, such as stress or anxiety. Therapists can guide individuals with these disorders through identifying and managing these factors.

Unconventional treatments can also be effective for parasomnias. For night terrors and sleepwalking, hypnotherapy has shown promise in reducing such episodes. During hypnosis, a trained therapist helps access a relaxed, focused state and introduces suggestions to reframe subconscious triggers. One study found that hypnosis reduced episodes of sleepwalking in participants over several weeks.[23]

Biofeedback and neurofeedback are techniques to train your brain to respond differently during sleep. Biofeedback uses sensors to monitor physical stress markers, such as heart rate, as you practice relaxation techniques. Neurofeedback tracks brainwaves and helps us retrain our brain's patterns, promoting better sleep stability. Both methods have shown potential for reducing sleepwalking and night terrors by calming overactive nervous systems.

Certain scents, such as lavender and chamomile, promote relaxation and may reduce the frequency of parasomnias triggered by stress. Use a diffuser with calming essential oils or apply them before bed. You can dab a few drops on your wrists, temples, or the back of your neck, or mix them with a carrier oil and gently rub them onto your chest or the soles of your feet before lying down. While this won't "cure" parasomnias, like many bedtime rituals, it can create a more soothing sleep environment. Also, some herbs have been traditionally used to promote relaxation and improve sleep quality. Valerian root and passionflower, which were mentioned as treatments for insomnia, have mild sedative properties that may calm the nervous system. Ashwagandha is an adaptogen that reduces stress and may help stabilize sleep cycles.

SLEEP PARALYSIS

Research suggests that up to 30 percent of the general population has experienced sleep paralysis—where you are fully conscious but unable to move your body or speak—at least once in their lifetime. The experience is often accompanied by intense fear or a sense of an ominous presence. While your breathing is not impaired, you may feel that you cannot breathe due to chest pressure. You may hallucinate and see shadows, figures, or lights; hear voices; or feel a sensation of being touched. Sleep paralysis can be caused by disrupted sleep patterns, sleep disorders such as narcolepsy, stress or anxiety, sleeping on your back, alcohol or drugs that disrupt REM sleep, and genetics. Essentially, sleep paralysis is the intrusion of REM sleep into wakefulness. There is a scientific explanation for it, but that may not be the entire story.

In Japanese culture, sleep paralysis is known as *kanashibari,* which translates to "bound in metal" or "tied down." The term connotes the sensation of being physically restrained, unable to move or speak. Historically and culturally, kanashibari has been associated with supernatural and spiritual deities that are part of Japan's rich tradition of folklore. It is thought that spiteful and vengeful spirits and ghosts (*yurei*) are responsible for restraining the individual or the paralysis is caused by a curse cast by someone who desires to exact revenge. Occasionally, kanashibari is thought to occur when an individual's spiritual defenses are weak, leaving them susceptible to these malevolent forces.

Scientifically, we now recognize that sleep paralysis occurs when REM sleep suddenly intrudes upon wakefulness as you're ready to enter sleep, something that usually happens because of fatigue, sleep deprivation, or keeping an irregular schedule. It is essentially an instance of REM rebound that occurs sooner than you'd like. You are awake but dreaming; REM, with its strange visual imagery, has encroached upon wakefulness. It is often frightening, as you're unable to signal that you can't move. It's more common for back sleepers. Interestingly, this phenomenon lasts seconds to mere minutes and can end if someone physically touches you.

Let me recount a bit of personal history that's still deeply etched in my consciousness. Approximately thirty years ago, while I was studying abroad at Meiji Gakuin University in Totsuka-ku, part of Yokohama in Kanagawa Prefecture, Japan, I had an experience of kanashibari that was infused with an uncanny metaphysical presence. I was living with a roommate in a small *apaato*: essentially a small apartment with one common room and a small kitchen and bathroom, no more than three hundred square feet.

Directly outside of this apaato stood a statue of the fox god Inari, the Shinto deity of rice, agriculture, and industry. Visitors to his modest shrine offered grains of rice and small coins for a promise of a better future, replete with wealth and success. Encountering the metal effigy of this fox-man, I'd immediately felt an affinity toward him. He towered high above me, at least ten feet in height, possibly taller, and his facial expression was stern yet somehow inviting. Fox-faced, with paws, he had the body of a man. He was caught in an awkward position: ready to pounce at a moment's notice, yet able to be restrained if his muscles contracted in time. It was this instantaneity, two divergent positions at once, that was so exciting. The digits of his metal paws were flexed, clawed but eroding, probably from decades of pigeon dung. This flaw highlighted his man-ness even more clearly. I empathized with this aspect of his mortality. Yet, he was still a god, this fox, and you only had to see him in his statuesque rawness to believe it. In this small village, the statue appeared to me like a hallucination of displacement—present and yet not fully there.

Even before the paralysis began, there was something uncanny about those nights in Japan: The air felt charged, the forest seemed alive with unseen presences, and sleep itself carried a strange, watchful quality.

One night, drifting to sleep, I felt Inari's presence in my room, his bronze fox head floating and bobbing high above me. Paralyzed, powerless, I could neither scream nor flee. Though it lasted only minutes, the vision felt endless, repeating itself as if it had always been there.

Later, drifting again into sleep, I saw not-quite-dead shadow people levitating me and trying to throw me off a two-story balcony. (They were unsuccessful, as I woke up before they performed their deed.) These two discrete episodes caused great nocturnal fear and dread in me whenever I'd try to sleep. Fearing Inari himself was somehow responsible for these episodes, I, like his Japanese worshippers, began offering him rice, with hope he'd disengage himself from my much-needed sleep.

I kept these experiences to myself for several years, until I matriculated at medical school at twenty-seven. Listening to a lecture on sleep physiology, I learned that what I'd experienced was a phenomenon of sleep paralysis, with its associated hypnagogic hallucinations. What I'd feared about and ascribed to Inari was nothing more than a misplaced remnant of a disrupted sleep "architecture." As adults, we undergo sleep cycles that normally start with stage one sleep and progress to more restful and deeper stages, culminating in rapid eye movement (REM) sleep.

Sleep paralysis occurs when REM sleep commences instantaneously as we're drifting to sleep, but not quite asleep. If REM is displaced onto the awake state, we're aware but paralyzed and susceptible to various dreamlike visual, auditory, gustatory, and tactile sensations. *Hypnagogia,* a term coined by the French scholar Alfred Maury, describes the transitional stage between wakefulness and sleep, while *hypnopompia,* its twin counterpart, named by the spiritualist Frederick Myers, describes the state leading out of sleep. Many kinds of hallucinations can occur during these liminal periods.

It's no wonder that sleep paralysis and its accompanying hallucinations have been associated with demons and hags, incubi and succubi. In African culture, the paralysis is referred to as "the witch riding our back," while in China it is known as the "ghost pressing on our body." Fascinatingly, Japanese people experience a higher frequency of sleep paralysis: There is a greater prevalence of narcoleptics in that country. (Sleep paralysis can be one of the criteria for the diagnosis of narcolepsy.[24])

Henry Fuseli's painting *The Nightmare* is considered a classic portrait of sleep paralysis. It wonderfully captures the hallucinatory quality of an incubus pressing on a body, the body of a woman, in this case, while she lies supine, presumably asleep, her arms dangling downward, powerless to flee. Even in 1781, Henry Fuseli got things right: He depicts the visual, often "demonic" hallucination that can be a part of sleep paralysis, the sense of suffocation, and the increased likelihood of experiencing it when sleeping face up, supine.

When I learned that irregular sleep schedules and sudden environmental changes are risk factors in experiencing ISP, I realized these factors likely brought me closer to my "demon" while I was in Japan, a demon that—in the end—was simply sleep debris, always arriving a little too early.

But was it *just* sleep debris? I share this experience some thirty years later because now that I'm a sleep physician and have a medical explanation for this phenomenon, the visceral nature of the moment still does not feel fully explained by the science. The vivid, terrifying nature invites interpretations that go beyond the physiological. Is it possible the supernatural quality of the experience lies in the universality and consistency of certain themes across cultures and histories, as well as its emotional and symbolic resonance? For example, across cultures, people report strikingly similar experiences during sleep paralysis, whether this is a malevolent presence in the room, the sensation of being pinned down or suffocated, or shadowy figures or otherworldly beings. These recurring elements could suggest a connection to the collective unconscious archetypes, as theorized by Carl Jung, or reflections of shared spiritual truths.

Similarly, experiences of sleep paralysis align closely with cultural myths, such as incubi and succubi in medieval Europe, kanashibari in Japan, the Old Hag in Newfoundland folklore, and shadowy figures described in modern alien abduction accounts. This enduring presence in folklore could imply an underlying metaphysical dimension or the existence of spiritual entities interacting with human consciousness.

Many of those who have experienced sleep paralysis describe a vivid, undeniable sense of being watched or visited during these episodes. I know that feeling well. During my own episode, the room seemed to breathe, and I could sense a presence hovering close, silent but intent. It was as if the night itself had become conscious and was studying me. Although this appears unlikely from a scientific stance, neuroscientific explanations, as illustrated by heightened amygdala activity in the brain, may not fully capture the intensity and certainty of these perceptions, leading some to suggest the involvement of spirits or inter-dimensional beings. Also, sleep paralysis occurs in a liminal state between sleep and wakefulness, which is often described as a "threshold" space in spiritual traditions. Such liminal states are often associated with increased spiritual or mystical access, where the boundaries between physical and metaphysical realms blur.

So, while my sleep paralysis can be explained scientifically, there was something there, on that night, that eluded neuroscience. Something that was ineluctably not tangible, something that could not be caught with the claws of science, as it were, evading it at every turn.

Those nights in Japan taught me that sleep isn't only a biological rhythm: It's a threshold. My paralysis could be explained by the brain's circuitry, yes; but what I felt was beyond explanation. In the stillness, something vast pressed close, something that science could describe but never touch. It was both terrifying and awe-filled, a reminder that not all mysteries are meant to be solved; some are meant to be felt.

From that moment, I began to see sleep not just as a process to understand but as a landscape to enter. The next part of this book is about that crossing: how to work with the forces that move through us at night, how to turn fear into curiosity, and information into experience. These practices—breath, attention, surrender—are my way of taking what I learned in that forest and shaping it into something luminous, a way of turning the science of sleep into the alchemy of awakening.

PART TWO

TRANSFORMATIVE SLEEP PRACTICES

4

TRANSFORMING THE MIND FOR REST

LONG BEFORE I UNDERSTOOD SLEEP, I LEARNED HOW DIFFICULT it is to trust the dark.

I was seven when I watched my grandfather kill a lamb. It happened in the courtyard of his home in Iran, the ground cracked and dry underfoot. He didn't say much. Just grabbed the lamb—small, trembling, almost weightless—and ended its life with one brutal, practiced move.

The smell of blood hit me first—sharp, metallic, alive. The lamb's body twitched once, then lay still, a dark, red stain spreading under it. I remember my twin sister squeezing my hand so tightly it hurt, both of us too stunned to move, too proud to cry in front of the adults.

That night, I didn't sleep. I lay stiff in the heat of the summer, blinking into the blackness, feeling as though something had splintered inside me. Sleep didn't feel safe anymore. Closing my eyes meant leaving myself exposed in a world that could change in a blink.

Even now, working as a sleep physician, I see traces of that instinct in many of my patients. Trouble sleeping isn't just about habits; it's also about fear and surrender. It's about the primal part of the brain that refuses to let its guard down. Sleep asks us to surrender, to give up control. And for some of us, including me, that doesn't come easily.

Through several decades of listening, observing, and learning from my patients, I've discovered that the way we think about sleep shapes the way we experience it. Sleep is not a passive state but an active exchange, a dialogue between the conscious and the unconscious, between the self and something greater and quite mysterious. Yet, so often, we approach sleep with resistance, frustration, or fear, layering it with unfounded beliefs that weigh it down. To invite sleep fully into our lives, we must first transform our relationship with it—a process as much spiritual as it is mental, a process akin to alchemy, turning that base metal into gold.

A NEW MODEL: COGNITIVE RESTRUCTURING

Most of what we know about treating insomnia still centers on cognitive behavioral therapy. It's a solid approach and often works wonders. But cognitive restructuring can help anyone rethink their relationship with sleep, whether insomnia is your issue or you just want to sleep better. But cognitive restructuring, reimagined as a form of inner alignment, is less about "fixing" sleep and more about learning to see it differently. It's an act of gentle alchemy, where rigid thoughts such as "I must sleep perfectly tonight" or "If I don't sleep, my day will be ruined" are softened, reexamined, and turned into something lighter, something more compassionate.

Imagine these thoughts as knots, tightened by worry or habit. Restructuring is the practice of loosening these knots, allowing the mind to breathe and flow freely. Instead of battling "perfect" sleep as an elusive goal that none of us will ever truly attain (even for me, as a sleep specialist), you can learn to view it as a gift, a natural rhythm that you are meant to align with, not control. You don't need to tighten your grip on sleep; you can simply let it be. Transforming a belief such as "I can't sleep" into "My body knows how to rest" invites trust and surrender to replace tension. This shift is not just mental. By reframing your thoughts, you don't just change your thinking; you acknowledge the larger truth that sleep is a space of grace, not a task to master. You allow it to be. You respect it, respect what it does for you without asking anything in return. Sleep can become a time when you relinquish the illusion of control and allow yourself to be carried by something deeper, something larger than you can ever conceive. It can be a reminder that, even in your vulnerability, you are held, embraced, and supported. In restructuring your thoughts, you are not simply finding better ways to think: You are honoring the sacredness of sleep as an act of renewal, connection, and trust.

To practice cognitive restructuring, take a moment to reflect on the beliefs you carry about sleep. Each night before you get into bed, consider your thoughts about sleep. Are they rigid, fearful, or rooted in frustration? Are you annoyed, inconvenienced, or dreading lying down? Write a few thoughts down, then gently question them by asking, "Is this thought serving me?" and "How else could I view this?" Reframe each thought with curiosity and kindness, creating space for a new narrative to take shape. This practice is not about perfection but about opening a door: to sleep, to rest, to the wisdom that lies within both. By framing cognitive restructuring as a spiritual realignment rather than a cognitive one, you can soften the edges of your mind and prepare for the renewal that only sleep can provide.

Your thoughts are the stories you tell yourself, and these thoughts can either help you embrace sleep or build bulwarks against it. Many of us carry beliefs about sleep that are shaped by fear, expectation, perfectionism, and the all-pervasive media—thoughts like, "I need at least eight hours to function during the day" or "If I don't sleep, my health will deteriorate, and my life will spiral downward." I've had these thoughts, too. So have most of us, at one time or another. These beliefs, though understandable, exacerbate anxiety and insomnia, pulling you away from your relationship with restful sleep.

This type of cognitive restructuring becomes a way to rewrite these stories, not by dismissing them but by compassionately reshaping them. It is the process of replacing rigid, fear-based thoughts with ones rooted in trust, curiosity, acceptance. For instance, the thought, "I'll never sleep well again, like the way I used to in my adolescent years," can be transformed into "Sleep is a process; my body and mind can find their way back to restful sleep at their own speed. It may take some time, but it will happen. I trust the process." This shift moves you from resistance to surrender, from control to connection.

At its heart, cognitive restructuring, when viewed in this light, is an invitation to practice surrender. Sleep, unlike many other aspects of life, cannot be forced or willed into being. It asks you to let go, to completely surrender, to trust in the body's innate wisdom to do what it needs to do, what it knows to do. Restructuring your thoughts aligns you with this principle, allowing you to release the need for control and embrace the mystery of sleep.

Think of the mind as a river, both turbulent and calm. During the day, the current rushes with thoughts, plans, and worries, carrying us forward. It is turbulent because it's active; it's overflowing with energy that is suitable for our daytime activities, but not conducive to sleep. This energy has potential, including the potential to disrupt our sleep. At night, we must allow this river to slow down, to find stillness in the turbulence that existed hours before. When unhelpful beliefs create turbulence: "I can't stop thinking" or "If I wake up at 3:00 a.m., my night and day will be ruined," they disturb this natural flow. By gently questioning these thoughts and offering kinder, more flexible alternatives, you have a chance to calm the waters and allow space for rest.

THE SPIRITUAL DIMENSIONS OF RESTRUCTURING

I have been hinting at it so far, but I want to emphasize how the practice of cognitive restructuring is not just a mental one. Inherent in the process are spiritual practices and principles such as mindfulness, inquiry, and self-compassion that can help you radically transmute your relationship with sleep.

Building mindful awareness, the act of seeing things as they truly are, is foundational to many spiritual practices. Cognitive restructuring begins with mindful awareness: noticing the unhelpful thoughts that arise around sleep without judgment. Simply recognizing these patterns is a step toward clarity. Once you are aware, you can engage in inquiry, a sacred process of questioning your thoughts. This is not about proving yourself wrong but about opening yourself to new possibilities, new threads, new viewpoints. An example of how to practice inquiry is to ask yourself, "Is this thought absolutely true?" "What is this thought protecting me from?" "What would it feel like to let this thought go?" In asking these questions, you allow space for gentler, more supportive beliefs and thoughts to emerge.

When you engage with yourself in this way, you start to rewrite your narrative from a place of compassion for yourself. The act of restructuring is not about forcing positivity that feels fake or ungenuine; rather, it's about finding thoughts that resonate with trust and an internal sense of well-being. For example, replace "I'm failing at sleep" with "Resting is enough for now; my body knows how to heal itself, in time." Transform "I can't function without eight hours of sleep" into "Every hour of rest supports my well-being, and I'm grateful for these hours." These reframed beliefs act as affirmations, aligning the mind with the restorative aspects of sleep. They are not meant to punish you for having "failed at sleep"; instead, they encourage you to think differently, to rest into the fact that your body knows what to do. This is not a test. This is not a performance. This is your body, and your body knows what to do, if you just allow it.

Sleep is a profound act of trust: trust in the body, in the natural cycles of life, in the unseen forces that guide us. By restructuring your thoughts, you align yourself with this trust, relinquishing the barriers that keep you from rest and sleep. It is ultimately a spiritual act of humility, recognizing that you do not need to control everything to be whole. You simply need to let go and surrender. You simply need to be.

In this way, such a restructuring becomes more than a technique: It becomes a path to honoring the sacred balance between effort and surrender, thought and silence, waking and sleeping. It is a practice of aligning the mind and spirit with the quiet, transformative power of rest. It becomes a beginning, each night, a renewal.

Incorporating this process into a nightly ritual can deepen its impact. Try this practice:

- *Create a sacred space.* Before bed, light a candle or dim the lights to signal a transition that you'll be surrendering. Sit quietly. Allow the busyness of the day to settle.
- *Journal your thoughts.* Write down any persistent beliefs or worries about sleep. For example, "I'm worried I won't fall asleep tonight and will be a wreck in the morning."
- *Gently question this premise and reframe it.* Reflect on each thought and ask, "How can I see this differently?" Then write a new narrative, one that feels genuine and honest.
- *Speak it aloud.* Read your reframed thoughts aloud as a form of affirmation, grounding them in your awareness.
- *Surrender.* Close your journal and take a deep breath. Imagine placing your reframed thoughts into a sacred vessel before you get into bed and let go into sleep.

SURRENDER: THE ART OF LETTING GO

As I tell my patients time and again, sleep is a paradoxical act. It requires us to do nothing, yet we often try too hard to make it happen. In our modern, productivity-driven world, this surrender—the act of simply letting go—feels unnatural. It feels passive. It feels weak. It feels selfish because we live in a world that values effort and strong work ethic. When we resist sleep, fight against it, we deny ourselves the rest we so deeply need. Sleep, then, isn't something we must conquer, something we must control in our tightest of grasps. It's something we want to invite into our life. This idea is simple, but it's profound and vital to our well-being and rest.

In our waking lives, we plan our days, chase goals, and manage every detail. We are always planning because we are concerned about the future that eludes us. We are always calculating because that is what we've been taught to do. We are always negotiating between what is required of us and what we desire. When bedtime arrives, most of us bring this same mindset to the pillow. But it's wrong. It's futile. We try to "force" sleep: lying in bed, counting hours, overanalyzing why it isn't arriving. We try to negotiate with sleep, just like in our waking lives. We demand things from it. We offer things in return for it. But sleep doesn't negotiate. It simply is. It offers its gift to us, asking nothing in return. But this exchange is too foreign for us, for us who are so used to negotiations, exchanges, a quid pro quo, a this for that, something for something else. But sleep wants nothing, desires nothing, and so we are baffled. We simply don't know how to respond to it. We want to control it. We want to make a deal with it, as we have been accustomed to do in all things. But sleep doesn't make deals. It simply gives without asking anything in return.

Sleep is the antithesis of control. It's not something we are able to will into existence. It simply is. Think of it as a delicate bird. We can't catch it by chasing it; we can only let it land when we're still. The more we grasp at sleep, the more it flies away. The key lies in releasing this control, in trusting our body's innate wisdom to carry us into rest, into sleep.

Surrendering to sleep may feel counterintuitive, especially in a culture that glorifies action and effort—indeed relishes it. But surrender, in this context, doesn't mean giving up; it means giving in. It's an act of trust, a relationship between us and sleep, of relinquishing the day's burdens and allowing ourselves to rest. Ask yourself: How often do you cling to the worries of the day, replaying conversations or planning for tomorrow? How often do you fret about the past, thinking about what went wrong, about your role in this debacle? These thoughts are like anchors, tethering you to wakefulness, to the day. To sleep, we must let go of the anchors and allow ourselves to drift into the unknown, into these mysterious, dark waters, which may be uncomfortable at first.

There's a deep wisdom in sleep that mirrors life itself: To truly experience peace, we must release what no longer serves us. The body already knows how to sleep. It's the mind that gets in the way and takes our sleep hostage. When we breathe naturally, we don't consciously think about each inhalation and exhalation. Our body takes care of it for us. Inhale, exhale. Air in, air out. Our sleep is no different. Trust your body to guide you. By relinquishing control, you create space for sleep to arrive naturally, gently, in its own time. But it will arrive, without any awareness. Wait for it. Because sleep simply is.

Surrendering to sleep doesn't happen instantly; it's a practice. Your mind needs to transition from wakefulness to rest, and the best way to do that is to embrace the art of letting go. Before bed, take a moment to consciously release the day. Reflect on what went well, acknowledge what didn't, and remind yourself that tomorrow is a new day, a new beginning, a tabula rasa. You can begin again and conquer a new day. Embrace imperfection. Stop pressuring yourself to have the "perfect" night of sleep, however that may be defined, whatever that might be for you. Some nights will be restless, and that's okay. Acceptance removes the anxiety that often perpetuates sleeplessness. Trust the process. Recognize that your body has a natural rhythm that you don't need to micromanage. Set the stage with a calming environment, but don't obsess about the outcome. Over the years, the patients who have really grasped this concept have found it to be one of the most helpful tools for improving their capacity for restful sleep.

Sleep teaches us a profound truth that is often difficult to grasp in our work-obsessed world: The harder we try, the further it slips away. This concept is foreign to us. Sleep cannot be forced; it must be allowed. And when we stop trying to control it, we discover sleep, like life, has a way of working itself out when we simply let go. In surrendering to sleep, we're not just resting our body; we're practicing a fundamental life skill. Letting go isn't just about sleep—it's about finding peace amid uncertainty, the uncertainty of life, the uncertainty of tomorrow. Sleep, in its quiet way, reminds us of the beauty of trust, the power of surrender, the art of simply being. So tonight, as you lie down, close your eyes and say to yourself: "I surrender. I trust my body. Sleep will come." Let yourself drift into the mystery known as sleep.

Surrendering to sleep requires courage. It's an act of faith in a world that often demands action. Staying awake can feel like holding on to the reins. It feels comfortable, familiar. Letting go, however, can feel like falling into the unknown, like flying, which I find terrifying but have begun to embrace. The act of letting go is deeply liberating. It reminds us that we don't need to carry the weight of the world with us every moment. Sleep is nature's way of telling us it's okay to rest, to pause, to let life continue without our constant input. Think of the way a child sleeps—in a car seat, on a parent's shoulder, or curled up in bed. They don't question whether sleep will come. They simply allow it. They let it be. There's a lesson here for us: Sleep doesn't require effort, only permission.

The philosopher Alan Watts said, "Muddy water is best cleared by leaving it alone."[1] The same can be said of the restless mind at bedtime. When we stop stirring the waters with our anxieties and plans, they settle on their own. Sleep doesn't arrive from solving every problem; it comes from stepping back and letting the mind rest in its natural state of stillness. Letting go doesn't mean silencing every thought; it means watching those thoughts float by, ungrasped. Like clouds drifting across the sky, they'll come and go without your intervention. Your job is not to control them but to trust that they will pass.

Surrendering to sleep is not a weakness; it's a profound strength. It's the moment we step out of our own way and allow life to unfold. It's a reminder that we are a part of a greater rhythm, that we are a part of a cycle of wakefulness and rest, action and stillness. In a world that celebrates productivity and control, surrendering to sleep is a quiet rebellion. It's a way of saying, "I trust the process. I trust myself. I trust that the world will continue to revolve as I let go. I'll simply be. I'm okay with that because that is natural."

BEFRIENDING FEAR

Sleep is one of the most vulnerable states we enter as humans. It asks us to relinquish control, lay down our defenses, and close our eyes to the world. For many, this surrender comes naturally. But, for others, sleep becomes a battleground, a place where fear lurks.

Many of my patients confess to something few admit out loud: They're afraid to fall asleep. Whether it's the fear of what dreams may bring, the fear of being unguarded, the fear of simply not sleeping at all, or the fear of sleep as death, being afraid of sleep can leave us restless. And yet, as the Buddhist philosopher Thich Nhat Hanh reminds us, fear is not an enemy but a companion to be spoken to and understood.[2]

At its core, sleep requires trust. We trust our bodies to keep breathing, our hearts to keep beating, and the world to keep turning while we rest and sleep. But for many, this trust is fragile. Fear tells us that if we let go, something will be lost: our control, our awareness, our safety, and, at the most extreme, our lives. Thich Nhat Hanh often speaks about fear as a product of attachment. We cling to our thoughts, our worries, and even our wakefulness because they feel familiar—like an old blanket that we cherish or a concert T-shirt we've worn for years, both symbols of safety and familiarity. However, embracing sleep feels like stepping into the unknown, and the unknown can be terrifying. Yet he teaches us that facing fear with mindfulness can transform it. Instead of resisting the fear of sleep, we can sit with it, acknowledge it, gently release it. He states, "The more we practice, the more we are gentle with our fear and are able to embrace it, the more the fear goes away."[3] So, it's a matter of getting to know our fear, understanding it, and, finally, letting it go.

To practice this, he suggests something as simple as focusing on the breath: *Breathing in, I calm my body. Breathing out, I let go.*[4] This mantra reminds us that fear cannot hold us if we stay anchored in the present. Sleep, like fear, becomes less overwhelming when we take it moment by moment, night by night.

The fear of sleep is universal, but the ways we understand it vary across cultures. In some traditions, sleep is seen as a liminal space, a borderland between life and death. Ancient Egyptians, for example, believed that sleep was a nightly encounter with the divine. They approached it with rituals and prayers, seeking protection from what lay beyond. In Japanese culture, sleep paralysis has long been associated with folklore about malevolent spirits. Even in Western culture, expressions such as "sleeping with one eye open" reveal the unease many feel about being defenseless in sleep. These cultural narratives remind us that fear in sleep is not just personal; it's woven into the human experience of vulnerability.

Philosophically, we can think of fear not as a barrier but as a gatekeeper. As the philosopher Søren Kierkegaard wrote, "Anxiety is the dizziness of freedom."[5] Fear, in this sense, arises when we stand on the edge of something unknown, something that requires us to surrender what we know for what might be. Sleep, with its stillness and mystery, embodies this leap. But fear also offers a profound opportunity. Thich Nhat Hanh teaches that fear is an instructor, pointing us toward what we most need to heal.[6] If we are afraid of sleep, what does that say about our relationship to trust? To stillness? To ourselves?

To find peace in sleep, we must approach fear not with resistance but with compassion. Instead of fighting the restless thoughts or the racing heart, we can acknowledge them with kindness: "I see you, fear. I know you're here. It's okay." This practice, rooted in mindfulness, allows fear to soften, to become more familiar. When we stop seeing fear as the enemy, it loses its grip, its power over us. Instead of a barrier to sleep, it becomes a companion—an indicator that we're standing at the edge of something important, something larger than we can imagine, something from which we can gather strength. As Thich Nhat Hanh suggests, "My dear, I'm not afraid of you. I'm not afraid of my fear."[7]

In her tenderly fierce book *The Places That Scare You*, Pema Chödrön discusses the concept of *bodhichitta*, which is the awakened heart-mind—rooted in compassion, courage, and deep vulnerability—that longs to relieve the suffering of all beings.[8] To her, bodhichitta isn't some lofty spiritual trophy; it's raw, exposed tenderness. It's the soft spot you instinctively want to protect when life cuts too close. It's the ache you feel when someone else is suffering. It's the willingness to stay present with that ache instead of bolting. In her view, bodhichitta is not cultivated by transcending human messiness; it's discovered right in the thick of it. The heartbreak, the uncertainty, the late-night anxiety spiral. If you've ever lain awake at 3:00 a.m. with your chest clenched and your thoughts racing, you've brushed up against the very terrain that bodhichitta asks us to stay with.

But we usually don't stay. Instead, we armor up. Enter the three lords of materialism—Pema's razor-sharp breakdown of how we spiritually bypass our discomfort. The lord of form says, "Buy this mattress, this supplement, this white noise machine, and you'll finally sleep." The lord of speech chimes in, "Read more. Understand your insomnia. Diagnose it. Fix it." And the lord of mind finishes the chant, "Control your mind. Meditate better. Think better." But, as Pema warns, all three may be just dressed-up avoidance strategies. These are all means of trying to conquer our restlessness rather than befriend it.

What if sleep issues aren't always a malfunction to be fixed but a messenger? What if insomnia is a kind of spiritual rebellion? What if it's our deeper self, refusing to be sedated by productivity, pharmaceuticals, or spiritual platitudes? Can we find the willingness to sit with the discomfort of not sleeping and feel what lies beneath it: the grief we haven't processed, the fear we've stuffed down, the tenderness we mistake for weakness? That's not an easy path. But maybe, it's the one that finally lets the nervous system unclench and allows sleep to come as an offering.

The teachings of the awakened heart, of bringing compassion to our experience, allow us to understand suffering (ours and others') with tenderness.[9] This may be our way out of poor sleep. As you lie in bed, quietly say to yourself: "May I be at ease. May others who are restless tonight also find peace." Let it be simple. If you're anxious, breathe into it. If you're wide awake, imagine all the other people in the world who feel just like you right now and send them a little compassion. This turns the struggle to sleep from a personal failure into a shared human moment.

Ultimately, sleep teaches us one of life's most profound lessons: how to rest in the unknown, how to blindly feel an unknown terrain. Every night, we close our eyes without knowing exactly what will come next. This act of surrender is not just physical, it's spiritual. It reminds us that we are part of something larger, something beyond our control. Fear will always be a part of the human experience, but it doesn't have to keep us awake. As Thich Nhat Hanh suggests, "Fearlessness is not only possible, it's the ultimate joy."[10] To sleep without fear is not to banish uncertainty, but to embrace it—to trust that even in the darkness, we are safe, protected.

Sit with fear. Listen to it. And then, when you're ready, let it go. Sleep is not the absence of fear; it's the quiet courage to rest in its presence and simply be.

5

DREAMS AS THE WINDOW INTO THE UNCONSCIOUS

I'VE HAD MANY VARIATIONS OF THIS DREAM: I'M STANDING IN A vast library, the Old Library at Trinity College in Dublin, Ireland, a place to which I traveled during my junior study abroad program at Leeds University in England. Its shelves stretch endlessly into the dark, into blackness, into a void that alarms me. The air is thick with the scent of aged paper and dust, a smell that I've always enjoyed, especially while visiting used bookstores. The only sound is the flickering of candlelight and the crackling of a fireplace somewhere. I reach for a book—a familiar one that I love to read: Roland Barthes's *Camera Lucida*. But when I open it, the pages are blank, white, erased of the words and images that I relish. Panicked, I flip through more books that I'm familiar with. Some are filled with words, but the sentences shift and dissolve before I can understand them. Others crumble into dust; some burn and shrivel in my hands.

A shadow moves at the end of the aisle. I know this figure, I tell myself, though I can't recall their name. "Hey, who are you?" I ask.

"Follow me," the shadow whispers, without revealing their name. I chase them, but the library begins to change, to shift—imperceptibly at first, but then markedly. The shelves warp, twisting into a labyrinth. The floor beneath me turns soft and starts to collapse and disintegrate. Somehow, I don't fall. But I'm so scared I begin to run. I forget why I'm running, though. And then a dirty mirror appears. I wipe it with my jacket; I see my own reflection, but it's not me. It's a stranger who looks like me, staring back with vacant, black eyes. A voice: my own, yet distant, echoes: *You're losing yourself, slowly, but you are losing yourself, don't you see that?* And then I wake up.

What could this strange series of events playing out like an exclusive screening of the latest David Lynch film possibly mean? What are dreams exactly, and what do they offer us? Why do they intrude into sleep, always forcefully, sometimes repetitively? Whether we ask for them or not, they are like a stranger knocking on our brain's door and letting themselves in without permission. They exist in our mundane world but are mystical, beyond our grasp. Are dreams repressed desires, as Sigmund Freud postulated? Are they expressions of the collective unconscious, a shared reservoir of archetypes and universal symbols, as Carl Jung believed? Could they be a narrative that the brain constructs from random brain activity during REM sleep, as neuroscientists John Allan Hobson and Robert McCarley suggest? Or, rather, are dreams a mechanism by which we can process emotions and solve problems we encounter during waking life, as the neuroscientist Rosalind D. Cartwright envisioned?

I would argue that dreams are all of those things and more. I don't believe that dreams can be relegated to one category. I think their origins and intentions are sundry. If dreams only mattered when we remembered them, most would be pointless because we forget nearly all of them. But that's the thing: Whatever dreams are doing, they're also doing it in real time: while we're asleep and the dream is happening, not just after we wake up. In this chapter, we'll explore competing ideas of why we dream and look at a variety of ways to work with our dreams to enhance our waking life—and even to help us prepare for death.

WHY WE DREAM

Across ancient cultures, dreams were seen as messages from the gods, glimpses of the future, or gateways to the spirit world. Each tradition wove its own rich mythology around them. But for the purposes of this book, we'll begin with the modern story of dream theory that really takes shape with Freud, who was the first to treat dreams as a window into the subconscious mind rather than messages from the divine. From a Freudian perspective, dreams fulfill repressed unconscious desires and resolve psychological conflicts. These desires cannot be shown outright but must be distorted and disguised to allow the dreamer to stay asleep. Thus, a residual dream censor, or the "dream-work (*Traumarbeit*)," distorts the normally repressed unconscious material for safe consumption. What we get, then, are two layers of the dream: the manifest content, which is a censored version that the dreamer experiences; and the latent content, the true meaning of the repressed wish that is often unacceptable or anxiety-provoking and must remain in the unconscious.

Jung, who was initially Freud's collaborator, eventually departed from Freud's theories, suggesting that dreams are expressions of the collective unconscious, a shared reservoir of archetypes and universal symbols that all humans tap into. The collective unconscious contains essentially all the inherited information of human experience—it's a storehouse that we are born with access to. It is not personal. It is related to all of humanity. Unlike Freud, Jung believed that dreams were not just repressed wishes but were tools for personal growth and self-integration.

Fritz Perls, the founder of Gestalt therapy, revolutionized the understanding of dreams in the 1950s and 1960s by shifting the focus from symbolic interpretation to direct experience. Perls believed that every part of a dream represents an aspect of the dreamer's own psyche. His approach involved "owning" the dream, that is, acting out different dream elements (even inanimate objects) to uncover unresolved emotions or conflicts.[1] For example, imagine a modern executive who keeps dreaming about a collapsing bridge. Rather than analyzing it as pure anxiety, a Gestalt approach would have them become the bridge and express what it feels like to "break under pressure." This active engagement turns the dream into a dynamic tool for growth.

Things diverge quite significantly in the understanding of dreams with the advent of the activation-synthesis theory, proposed by the psychiatrists and neuroscientists John Allan Hobson and Robert W. McCarley in 1977, which dominated the dream landscape for some time.[2] In short, the theory proposes that dreams result from random brain activity during REM sleep and have no subconscious meaning—a hypothesis that, in one blow, obliterated nearly one hundred years of approaching dreams as messages from the subconscious. In the activation-synthesis theory, the activation phase involves the brainstem stimulating the cortex, creating random images and thoughts. It is followed by the synthesis phase, where the brain attempts to create a coherent narrative from these fragmented signals. These two phases create the dream as we know it. Essentially, said Hobson and McCarley, there is nothing more going on than the brain trying to make sense of senseless material.

Meanwhile, in 2000, the Finnish psychologist Antti Revonsuo suggested dreaming, or at least nightmares, simulate threatening events to prepare us for the real thing. In a sense, you rehearse threats in your dream to practice staying alive in a crisis. Repeated simulations of such events, from an evolutionary perspective, would offer a selective advantage in terms of a faster response time to, or easier detection of, a threatening event.[3]

Revonsuo and several other researchers expanded this hypothesis in 2015 and proposed a social stimulation theory of dreaming, where dreamers maintain and practice various evolutionarily important functions of social perception and social bonding. When we dream, as this theory suggests, the brain recreates social situations—arguments, reconciliations, alliances—as a kind of overnight rehearsal. By running these scenarios, our minds keep social perception and bonding skills sharp, helping us navigate real-world relationships more effectively, just as it may have helped our ancestors in the past.[4] In this case, dreams function as a kind of mental rehearsal for social survival, fine-tuning our ability to read social cues, predict others' behaviors, and handle tricky situations.[5]

Think about a time you had a dream about a difficult conversation, perhaps confronting a friend, asking for a promotion, or handling an argument. The next day, when faced with a similar real-world scenario, you might feel more prepared, as if you've already "practiced" the moment in your sleep. Athletes, performers, and even students cramming for exams often experience dreamlike rehearsals where they perfect skills or manage stress, which can enhance confidence and performance in waking life. Similarly, a person who frequently dreams about navigating social interactions might become more adept at handling real-world relationships, whether it's smoothing over workplace tensions or strengthening personal bonds. In a way, our dreaming brains act like an advanced social training ground, constantly refining our ability to thrive in human interactions.

Rosalind D. Cartwright's hypothesis of why we dream blends the science and spiritual aspects of dreaming in a way that makes the most sense to me. Her theory emphasizes a dream's role in emotional regulation and problem-solving. In her view, dreams serve as a way for processing and integrating emotional experiences, particularly during times of stress. Her research also shows that dreams help individuals work through unresolved emotions and conflicts, allowing the mind to adapt and prepare for forthcoming challenges. Similarly, the emotional tone of dreams can influence waking life and maintain a psychological balance that is productive and healthy. In short, Cartwright believed that dreams regulate our emotions over the course of the night, without our conscious awareness. Dreams direct us to well-being by allowing us to process our emotions in a safe space.

While Freud and Cartwright explored dreams through the lens of meaning and emotion—Freud seeing them as disguised wish fulfillment and Cartwright seeing them as nightly therapy for mood regulation—newer models approach dreaming as a function of the brain's intrinsic networks. The NEXTUP model (Network Exploration to Understand Possibilities)—a term coined by sleep and dream researchers to describe how the brain uses dreams—belongs to this modern lineage, shifting the focus from interpretation to neural exploration. It suggests that the dreaming brain is rehearsing possibilities, testing connections and creative solutions beyond waking constraints. In this way, it extends the history of dream theory from symbolic narrative to dynamic neuroscience. It's like our mind is delving through old files and suddenly noticing patterns it missed before, turning scattered memories into fresh insights.[6]

What makes NEXTUP so relevant is how it shifts our view of dreams. Instead of being meaningless or purely symbolic, dreams may serve a vital adaptive function by helping us mentally rehearse, emotionally process, and even prepare for future decisions by creating fresh connections between old and new memories. That strange dream about missing a flight or arguing with your supervisor? It may be your brain pressure-testing scenarios that feel emotionally charged or uncertain. In essence, then, dreams could be one of the brain's most powerful tools for navigating the complexities of life—if we learn how to listen to them.

REMEMBERING YOUR DREAMS

When I meet people for the first time and tell them that I'm a sleep specialist, one of the first questions I get is, "Why can't I remember my dream a few minutes after I wake up, although I remembered it seconds after awakening? Why do they evaporate so quickly?" That's a very perceptive question and the answers are quite interesting.

Dreams can feel incredibly vivid while you're in them, yet within a few minutes of waking up, they're almost impossible to recall. One reason is that dreams primarily occur during REM sleep, a stage where your brain isn't set up to create strong, lasting memories. Instead, it's busy processing emotions and sensations in a way that's quite different from how it handles daytime information. Another reason involves the way your brain consolidates memory. During sleep, especially REM sleep, your hippocampus, the part of the brain responsible for forming new memories, is less active when it comes to capturing the ephemeral details of your dreams. It shows reduced involvement in memory replay compared to during NREM sleep. This means that even if the dream feels intense or emotional now, it doesn't get the full "storage treatment" it needs to be recalled later.

Then there's the matter of brain chemistry. During REM sleep, when most vivid dreaming occurs, norepinephrine is almost entirely switched off, which is unusual because it's normally active when we're awake and storing memories. At the same time, acetylcholine levels are elevated, which helps to create the vivid, emotional, and often bizarre qualities of dreams. But without norepinephrine, the brain doesn't flag those experiences as "important to remember." So, when you wake up and norepinephrine floods back in, it's too late; the dream wasn't tagged for storage, and it fades like steam off a mirror. It's not that the dream didn't happen; it just never made it to the filing cabinet.

Yet another reason that dreams fade so fast is the nature of the dreams themselves. Dreams often don't follow the logical narrative structures that our waking mind prefers. Their bizarre, fragmented qualities make them harder to encode into long-term memory. And when we do wake up, our brains immediately switch gears to focus on the real world—on tasks, plans, and even worries about the day ahead—pushing those ephemeral dream details further into the background. There's also the matter of sleep inertia, that groggy period right after waking up when the brain is transitioning from sleep to full alertness. This transitional state can interfere with your ability to transfer the delicate impressions of dreams into long-term memory. All these elements together create a quiet convergence, ensuring that by morning, your dreams are like gossamer, and they have already begun to slip away.

If you want to start using dreams as tools for insight and healing, the first step is to practice remembering your dreams. The easiest way to do that is by writing them down as soon as you wake up. Keep a notebook by your bed and jot down whatever you remember, even if it's just a single image, word, or feeling. Or you might consider making a voice memo or using a dream app that allows you to make an audio recording of your dream. Some apps will transcribe and even analyze your dream for you. At first, it might feel like you're grasping at straws trying to remember details, but with practice, your dream recall will improve. Don't worry about making sense of it right away; just focus on capturing the details, however limited or bizarre they may be.

One way to increase the chance of remembering your dreams is to remain still and keep your eyes closed when you first wake up. In this way, you are only half-removed from your dream world. (Creating an audio recording can help with this so you don't need to turn on the light to get your glasses or a pen and journal.) Try to stay relaxed because becoming tense or overexcited may interfere with recalling the dream images. Prompt yourself with various, basic questions: "Where was I?" "What did I want?" "What was the dilemma?" "How did it resolve?" These answers will aid you in staying in your dream longer, so you can recall it more clearly.

Dreamwork can also begin before your head hits the pillow. By setting intentions for both your sleep and the dreams that follow, you can create a purposeful connection between your waking life and the rich, symbolic world of the unconscious. Think of it as priming the mind for exploration—a practice that not only deepens your dreamwork but also enhances your rest. You are allowing your mind the freedom to explore, to navigate the expansive neural networks of the cortex and limbic system. Use intention to prime your mind, intently and effectively, and your dream recall is likely to increase.

Dreams don't emerge in isolation; they reflect and interact with our waking thoughts, emotions, and experiences. By consciously setting intentions, we can guide our dreams and steer our unconscious toward themes or questions we want to explore: "Am I working in the right field of work?" "Do I want a family?" "What do I really want from life?" A clear intention also signals to your mind that dreams are valuable, increasing the likelihood of remembering them. In addition, aligning your mental focus with rest can soothe the mind, making it easier to fall and stay asleep. Remember: Intentions are not demands; they are kind invitations. You can come as you are, as you were. The unconscious thrives on curiosity and openness, not rigid control.

Remember also that you want to be as fluid as possible. Reflect on your purpose. Ask yourself: "What do I hope to gain from tonight's dreams or rest?" Your purpose can be specific or broad, such as: "I want insight into my feelings about a career change." If your focus is on rest, your intention might be as simple as: "I will allow my body and mind to rejuvenate tonight. I will allow my dreams to take me there."

I've mentioned pre-bed rituals several times in the book so far, and I'll go into creating one more deeply in appendix B. So it shouldn't come as a surprise that before-bed rituals can help with dream recall.

A consistent ritual anchors your intention and prepares your mind for sleep. Wind down by dimming the lights, turning off screens, and engaging in calming activities such as reading or journaling. Affirm your intention by saying it out loud or writing it in a dream journal. Adding in practices such as deep breathing, progressive muscle relaxation, or gentle stretching can also help. Repetition is key here. Over time, as your bedtime ritual becomes natural, it becomes a cue for your mind to align with your goals for the night.

Visualization practices can also enhance your intention-setting process. As you lie in bed, imagine yourself entering a dream world that's rich and overflowing with symbols and meaning. Imagine your dreams bringing clarity, healing, or creativity. Pair this with affirmations like: "I will wake refreshed and remember what I need to" or "The dream will guide me to a place where I want to be, where I need to be."

The unconscious mind is like a wise, enigmatic partner. Treat it with respect and curiosity. Nourish it. Converse with it. Before sleep, ask it a question or make a request. You can ask questions such as "What message do I need to hear tonight? Why?" or "Show me an image that will guide my next steps." Be patient. Answers may not come immediately or in obvious ways. Dreamwork is a dialogue; it's not like the transactions we are used to in waking life. You will not get a yes-or-no answer to your questions. The answers will be long-winded, often rambling and confusing, and it'll be up to you to sort them out. Dreams will show you something, but you must parse the answers out yourself.

The benefits of intention setting go beyond dreaming. Setting intentions trains your mind to approach rest and personal growth with purpose. It fosters mindfulness, deepens self-awareness, and strengthens the connection between your conscious and unconscious selves. Through consistent intention-setting, you'll find that your dreams become vivid, meaningful, and accessible. And even on nights when dreams escape you, the very act of aligning your focus with rest brings its own reward: a calmer, more centered waking life.

The beauty of dreamwork is that it encourages self-awareness and emotional healing in a gentle, noninvasive way. You don't have to force anything. You don't have to mold anything. Your subconscious will bring up what you're ready to face, one step at a time. By engaging with your dreams, you might find that not only does your sleep improve, but you also feel more in tune with yourself. And when you start to approach sleep and dreams as a sacred space for insight and renewal, they become less of a struggle and more of a gift.

WAYS TO WORK WITH YOUR DREAMS

Once you have improved your dream recall and are remembering more of your dreams, you can begin to work with them. There are many ways to approach dreamwork. I introduce several of them in what follows, but there is no one-size-fits-all. If you find yourself drawn to a particular approach, dive deeper and explore how it can help you understand your nighttime visions. Here are a few things to consider as you begin:

- *Think of your dream as a mirror.* Have you ever had a dream that left you feeling unsettled or deeply moved, even if it didn't make logical sense? Or a dream from which you didn't want to awaken because it was really that good, that fulfilling? Dreams are like a mirror, reflecting your innermost fears, desires, and emotions in symbolic form.

  When I was going through a particularly stressful period at work, when my responsibilities were accruing and no one was there to assist me, I kept having a recurring dream about running late for an exam I hadn't studied for or didn't know I had. At first, I brushed it off as random stress. But when I started journaling about it, I realized the dream was highlighting my fear of being unprepared—not just at work, but in other areas in my life. This anxiety also manifested itself in other dream scenarios such as being enclosed in an elevator that was falling precipitously and driving a car maniacally off a cliff. The scenarios were all different, but the emotions they elicited were similar: that of anxiety. So, it wasn't necessarily about understanding what the images signified exactly, but rather about the feelings they projected.

Dreams often bring to light what we might not be consciously aware of, giving us a chance to process and release it. Acknowledging that fear allowed me to address it head-on, and, interestingly, those types of dreams stopped appearing. My sleep also surprisingly improved.

- *Look for patterns.* Over time, start reviewing your dream journal to look for recurring themes, symbols, or emotions. One dream might feel random, but recurring symbols, emotions, or scenarios often form important themes. Do you keep dreaming about water? Flying? Being chased? These symbols often carry personal or universal meanings. For example, dreaming about water might symbolize emotions or change, while flying could represent freedom or a desire to escape. Ask yourself: "What is the common thread among these dreams? What's happening in my waking life that might relate to these themes?" You might even use technology to help find patterns and identify the frequency of people, places, or emotions in your dreams.
- *Explore emotions.* Dreams are less about what happens and more about how they make you feel. The narrative just propels the dream along, but it's the essence of the dream that's important. Instead of getting hung up on the details, pay attention to the emotions your dreams evoke, such as fear, joy, excitement, frustration, or sadness, and ask yourself if these emotions are showing

up in your daily life. I once consulted with a patient who dreamed of standing on a stage, unable to speak. After some reflection, she realized the dream mirrored her fear of expressing herself in a difficult family situation. Once she worked on finding her voice in her waking life, her sleep improved, and the dream stopped recurring. It wasn't the dream content that mattered but rather the emotion of fear when she was alone on that stage.

- *Use active imagination.* If a dream leaves you feeling curious or unresolved, you can work with it consciously through active imagination. This involves revising the dream in your mind when you are awake and "interacting" with it. For instance, if you dreamed of being lost in a forest, find a quiet place to sit and imagine returning to that forest. What happens if you ask for guidance or follow a path? What if you decide to remain in this forest to see if anyone will find you? If there was a person in your dream, visualize them and ask them questions like, "What do you need from me?" "Why are you in my dream?" "What is your purpose here?" This technique strengthens connections between the logical and emotional parts of the brain, helping you extract deeper insights and process emotions tied to the dream.

A Neuro-Jungian Approach

Dreams are more than random bursts of neural activity; they are bridges between the biological rhythms of the brain and the symbolic language of the psyche. A neuro-Jungian approach blends modern neuroscience with the timeless insights of Carl Jung to explore not just how dreams emerge, but why they matter for personal growth. By understanding both the mechanisms and meanings of dreams, you can engage with them more deeply and uncover layers of insight.

The brain's default mode network (DMN)—a system activated

during rest, creativity, and introspection—plays a central role in producing dreams. This network weaves together memories, emotions, and symbols, giving rise to the surreal yet meaningful narratives we experience each night. Jung viewed dreams as messages from the unconscious, filled with archetypal symbols and personal material that guide us toward individuation, or becoming our truest selves. A neuro-Jungian perspective combines these ideas: Dreams are both neurobiological processes and gateways to self-discovery.

Archetypes are universal patterns—like the hero, the shadow, and the wise elder—encoded in our collective unconscious, which Jung described as a shared psychological inheritance. From a neuroscientific viewpoint, these archetypes may correspond to deeply ingrained neural circuits shaped by evolution and culture, influencing how we perceive and interpret the world. Certain dream themes are nearly universal, reflecting how these archetypes work in our subconscious thoughts, fears, and desires. Here are some common examples:

- *Falling.* Dreams of falling often symbolize a feeling of being out of control—in your career, relationships, or personal life. If you're experiencing stress or anxiety, your brain may translate that helplessness into a free fall. Sometimes, though, the fall feels peaceful, signaling a need to let go and surrender to something new. Falls aren't necessarily "bad"—sometimes we need to fall to rise again and create a better version of ourselves.
- *Being chased.* Dreams of being chased are another common experience, often signaling avoidance. Whether it's a faceless figure, a wild animal, or something supernatural, the feeling is the same: You must get away or face some consequence. Ask yourself: "Is there something in my waking life I'm running from—a difficult conversation, a responsibility, or a part of myself I'd rather not confront?"

- *Flying.* Flying dreams are probably the most exhilarating, especially if you're soaring effortlessly. These often reflect feelings of freedom, confidence, or a desire to escape reality. If you're struggling to stay airborne, though, you may feel held back from achieving your goals. The context always matters.
- *Losing your teeth.* Losing your teeth in a dream is one of the most unsettling experiences. Teeth symbolize power and confidence, so losing them often represents insecurity, embarrassment, or fear of aging. It can also be tied to transitions, like a major life change or a new job. Some cultures see this dream as a sign of personal growth—shedding the old to make way for the new.
- *Public nakedness.* Being naked in public is the ultimate vulnerability dream. It often points to insecurity or fear of being exposed, literally or figuratively. Maybe you're in a new situation where you feel unprepared, or you're afraid others will see something you're trying to hide. If no one in the dream seems to notice, your fears of embarrassment may be exaggerated. If everyone is staring, it could reflect anxiety about judgment or feeling out of place.
- *Car out of control.* Losing control of a car is another anxiety-fueled dream. Driving often symbolizes control over your life's direction. If the car is out of control, you might feel powerless in some area of your life. If someone else is driving, ask yourself: "Who is making decisions for me, and am I comfortable with that?"

Ultimately, dream interpretation is not an exact science, and symbols deemed universal may mean something different to you. Some dreams are random, while others carry deep personal significance. The key is to focus on your emotions during the dream—fear, excitement, anxiety, relief—and connect those feelings to your current life. Each symbol in your dream carries a unique meaning that's personal to you.

Don't rely solely on generic interpretations; look for connections that arise from your own unconscious mind.

Identify the emotional core of your dream, as this is often the glue that ties the narrative together. Ask yourself: "What emotions stood out in this dream? Do these emotions mirror anything I'm experiencing in my waking life?" For Jung, emotions in dreams were vital clues to unresolved conflicts or desires. Neuroscience agrees: Emotional centers such as the amygdala are highly active during REM sleep, amplifying the emotional tone of dreams.

Dreams rarely speak in plain language. Instead, they use symbols, metaphors, and archetypes. While some may have shared meanings, as I just shared above, what a symbol means to you personally will always be more important in understanding your dreams. For example, a snake might mean danger to one person but signal transformation and healing to another. A dream about being lost in a forest may connect to the archetype of the hero's journey, symbolizing a need for self-discovery, or it could reflect grief over a recent loss. An elderly figure could represent a wise mentor or a fear of aging. Remember: It's your personal associations with these symbols that make their meaning clear. (We'll explore this more later in this chapter.)

Dreams often feel illogical because they use symbolic, not linear, language. Neurologically, the right hemisphere (creativity and intuition) dominates during dreaming, weaving symbols and metaphors, while the left hemisphere (logic and structure) is less active. That's why dreams feel fragmented but rich with meaning—they bypass rational filters and speak directly to your emotional core.

A neuro-Jungian approach doesn't prioritize neuroscience over meaning or vice versa. Instead, it recognizes that dreams are where biology and psyche meet. Understanding how the brain creates dreams helps us appreciate the practical mechanisms behind them, while Jung's insights show us why they matter for personal growth. So, the next time you dream, don't dismiss it as random or meaningless. See it as a gift from your brain and psyche, inviting you to explore, heal, and transform.

SOFIA'S DREAM

Let's see how this approach works by looking at the experience of a patient of mine. Sofia,[7] a twenty-nine-year-old graphic designer, was feeling stuck in her career. She was working for a well-known tech company but often felt intimidated by the "bro culture" that pervaded the workplace. Although she loved her work, she avoided taking on more creative, high-stakes projects for fear of failure in a company that was overrun and dominated by men. She began to have a recurring dream that made it difficult for her to stay asleep. That's when she consulted me.

In her dream, she's walking through a dimly lit corridor with countless doors on either side. She stops at one door that feels important, but it's locked. She jiggles the handle, pushes on the door, and even tries peering through the keyhole, but it won't open. She would like to kick the door open with all her force and energy but decides against it. After all, people could be watching her and she must preserve decorum. *There must be a reason this door is closed*, she thinks. But she feels a mix of frustration, curiosity, and fear. Suddenly, she hears a voice behind her say, "You're not ready. You never were. Go back, girl! You don't belong here." She would then awaken with her heart racing, unable to breathe and unable to return to sleep.

One can approach this dream through dreamwork in various ways. Sofia's first step was to write down the dream immediately upon waking. In this way, she captured not just the events, but also the emotions (frustration, curiosity, fear, resentment) and any sensory details (the dim lighting, the sound of the voice).

I then asked her to engage with the symbols in her dream. In dreamwork, symbols are rarely literal; they're unique to the dreamer. I recommended that she ask questions like, "What does the locked door remind me of in my waking life? Is it constraining? Do I want to readily escape it?" "What am I afraid to open or explore?" "What might I gain or lose if I walk through it?" For Sofia, the door could symbolize her creative ambitions or her fear of taking risks in her burgeoning career. The voice saying "You're not ready" may represent an internalized critic from past experiences, perhaps a parent, teacher, or her own perfectionism that was preventing her from doing what she truly desired or needed.

I urged Sofia to implement active imagination, a key Jungian technique, which would allow her to continue the dream's narrative in her waking state. She could close her eyes, visualize the dream scene, and mentally reenter it. Sofia might imagine asking the voice "Why am I not ready?" or she could walk further down the corridor and try other doors or see what other elements were there that she did not recollect at the time of her dream. She could visualize herself finding a key, picking the lock, or pushing through the door. These exercises would allow her to engage directly with her subconscious and explore possibilities the dream left unresolved.

I also encouraged Sofia to treat elements of the dream (e.g., the door, the voice) as parts of herself and hold a conversation with them, extending the concept of active imagination. For example, she could journal the responses as she was speaking to the door or with the voice. Sofia could ask the door, "Why are you locked?" and the door could respond with, "I'm waiting for you to gather courage." Or Sofia may ask the voice, "Why do you think I'm not ready?" and the voice could reply with, "You doubt yourself more than you should. The door will open when you believe you can walk through it." This technique would allow her to integrate conflicting parts of her psyche to gain clarity into her inner struggles. She would be actively engaging with the characters and aspects in her dream to formulate problems, desires, solutions.

Although Sofia gained significant insight into her recurring dream, this wouldn't produce any significant results in her waking life unless she takes conscious action. In other words, dreamwork is incomplete if we don't act on the insights we have. For Sofia, the dream may be urging her to face her fears and take creative risks. She may take this on by accepting a small, but challenging, project at work. Or she might identify a skill or resource she feels she needs to cultivate to "be ready" and work toward it by taking a specialized course or seeking a mentorship.

From a clinical perspective, I was able to work with Sofia on this dream and address the anxiety and fear surrounding the door. Once she realized that she was anxious and fearful of taking on bigger projects and this was her obstacle, she spoke with the project manager of her team to express interest in taking on a larger role in the artificial intelligence program that they were spearheading. She was put in charge of a specific portion of that project, and she flourished. Her excitement became evident, and she began connecting with the others on her team, discovering that she belonged and that this was not the "bro culture" she had imagined. In this way, a dream that was initially rooted in anxiety and fear allowed her to explore its transformative potential and make her push through that door.

Sofia's dream didn't just reveal her fear; it gave her a map. That's the power of dreamwork: What seems like an obstacle is often an opportunity or a threshold. When we're willing to look closer, our dreams can nudge us toward growth we didn't know we were ready for.

Identify Your Own Symbology

Dreams speak to us from a place that is both intimate and foreign. From a neuroscientific perspective, they arise from multiple areas of the brain, including the limbic system and the cortex. The pons, thalamus, amygdala, and hippocampus all contribute to the integrity of the dream, while also processing emotions and integrating past experiences into dream content. But while neuroscience explains the mechanisms of dreaming, personal meanings still abound in dreams. Think of it this way: While the brain acts as the producer and technical apparatus of the dream (as in a film), the actual film is more personal and is supported by what you supply (the script, actors, settings, and so forth). This is highly idiosyncratic and makes working with your own dreams an important component to understanding their messages.

Earlier in this chapter, I discussed how certain motifs such as flying or losing teeth are understood to have a universal meaning. Carl Jung believed the collective unconscious, a deep layer of shared human psyche, carries shared memories, myths, and archetypes that are consistent across cultures and generations. You can think of it like the "greatest hits" of human symbolism. Across history, in different societies, certain dream symbols tend to appear repeatedly. For example, water often signifies emotions, the subconscious mind, or transformation, while flying symbolizes freedom, escape, and enlightenment. However, there are many examples where the same symbol means different things. In some cultures, snakes signify healing and wisdom, while in others, they point to danger and betrayal.

In essence, not all symbols mean the same thing to everyone. It's really our personal experiences, culture, and language that shape how we interpret a dream. Let's say you were bitten by a dog as a child like I was. In the United States, dreaming of a dog might be said to symbolize loyalty and companionship. But for me, it can signal fear. I like dogs when I'm awake, but in dreams, they trigger anxiety in me. Similarly, water, which typically symbolizes peacefulness and calm, may signify something terrible if you had a near-drowning experience.

One of my clients would often dream of being at her aunt and uncle's home. She didn't understand why—it was a nice enough place, with some fond memories from childhood, but she had never lived there and wasn't really in touch with them as an adult. After working with her dreams for some time, she realized that even though she was dealing with her father passing away and her mother being in advanced stages of Alzheimer's, she never dreamed of her own childhood home. It turns out her psyche was using her aunt and uncle's house to stand in as a safe place for processing her grief and loss.

Dream symbols need to be placed in context based on you and what is occurring in your life at that moment. This is the coolest thing about dreams: They form their own personalized language, their own dream dictionary, over time, for you. Your brain picks up on things that are meaningful to you, not just what's written in a dream dictionary or offered up from a dream interpretation app.

Rather than relying on someone else's dream symbolism, you can create your own dream dictionary. After you have journaled or recorded somewhere between thirty to fifty dreams, go through them and analyze them by picking out the symbols that stood out to you. (Some apps will do this for you, and basic AI programs excel at this as well.) For example, in your dream, you may have had images of a house, water, a car, emotions, friends, and so forth. Write down anything that is obvious to you and then begin grouping them into bundles. If you dreamed of water, ship, and fish, these can be categorized together. You can then link this group of images to emotions that you experienced, such as peace and tranquility, if the sea for you has been a symbol of freedom and movement. Some of these symbols may change meaning over time depending on where you are in your life, but this is another wonderful dimension of using dreamwork to understand yourself and track your own personal and spiritual development. There is no right or wrong answer. Your aim is to question, analyze, and grow. The dreams are there to serve you, not the other way around. This is not a test. You're using your dreams as a platform to grow, to face the dilemmas of your daily life, and to succeed.

MY DREAM

Let's see how working with a neuro-Jungian approach to dreamwork combined with an understanding of my own symbology helped me to understand the dream that I recounted at the beginning of the chapter. This dream of being lost and disoriented in a vast library, and losing access to books and words in them, speaks directly to an anxiety that I've had for quite some time: losing access to my mind and becoming demented. I have family members with dementia, who were all high-functioning and well educated and now behave like children who need assistance with everything. This thought frightens me and is often reflected in my dreams. I worked through this dream with a psychologist versed in dreams, and together the analysis has given me a deeper understanding of my fears and how to act on them in my waking life.

The vast, endless library symbolizes accumulated knowledge and identity, while its stretch into the darkness and void represents my anxiety over the unknown or the fear of losing access to my intellect, past, or awareness. It evokes my fear of losing access to the knowledge that lies before me, something that I can't ever retrieve! The scent of old books is comforting to me, representing a deep connection to learning, nostalgia, and my core identity as a scholar and lover of learning. The scent is intimate: It takes me back to a place that I can associate with home, satisfaction, relaxation. The familiar book turning blank signifies a loss of meaning or a struggle to hold on to a sense of self. Books often symbolize personal beliefs, identity, and memory. Their disintegration suggests a disconnectedness from oneself.

In shadow work (which we will talk about in chapter 7), a shadowy presence often represents a repressed or hidden part of oneself. I, the dreamer, know this figure but can't recall their name, suggesting that this part of myself was once known but has been buried or forgotten. That whispered invitation to follow hints at confrontation with the unconscious, an opportunity for self-discovery. The shifting library mirrors the instability of myself, as though the mind is restructuring itself in ways that I can't fully control. In a similar manner, the labyrinth represents feeling lost within my own psyche or undergoing a transformation that feels disorienting and frightening.

A floor turning soft suggests anxiety, instability, or a fear of losing control. The fact that I don't fall implies resilience, even in the face of this uncertainty. Mirrors in dreams often symbolize self-perception, identity, and truth. The stranger with vacant eyes could represent my unconscious fears, suppressed emotions, or an unfamiliar version of myself—a version I'm afraid of becoming. The whispered phrase "You are losing yourself" suggests an inner warning. It might indicate the ego struggling to maintain a coherent self-image amid deep psychological changes or personal turmoil. In short, the accumulated symbolisms in this dream reflect my fears and anxiety of developing cognitive impairment, like my family members have later in their lives. It's a call to understand this anxiety and do something about it, especially in the context of the traumatic brain injury in that car crash several decades ago. In waking life, that might mean engaging in regular neurological checkups and cognitive screening, practicing mindfulness and cognitive exercises to strengthen attention and memory, and exploring therapy to work through the underlying fear. It might also involve cultivating acceptance by acknowledging uncertainty while focusing on daily habits that support brain health, such as restorative sleep, physical activity, and meaningful connection.

This neuro-Jungian, symbol-based approach may feel familiar. If you've engaged in any therapy or dreamwork, you may have encountered the process of looking for the bridges between psyche and science, myth and mind. Yet dreamwork can move beyond interpretation into something more intimate: an act of participation. When we step inside the dream rather than stand apart from it, the images begin to breathe, becoming a living language. The following sections will show you how.

Lucid Dreaming

Imagine a dream where you realize you're dreaming, yet the world around you feels vivid and real. You can fly, explore your unconscious, or simply observe the landscape of your mind. This is the art of lucid dreaming, a state where the dreamer is aware of dreaming and can sometimes influence the dream's content.

For centuries, lucid dreaming has fascinated spiritual seekers, psychologists, and scientists alike, with its unusual combination of rest, creativity, and self-awareness. While often perceived as a whimsical curiosity, lucid dreaming holds profound potential for improving sleep quality and offering personal insight. I've also found that lucid dreaming allows for a sense of control that people often find missing from their lives. Some of my patients have told me that they're interested in lucid dreaming because it allows them to be in control of things that they otherwise cannot be in their waking lives. They've felt powerless, weak, lacking in creativity, lethargic, listless. Lucid dreaming became a way for them to take control of situations in their dream lives. And when they felt comfortable in their dream lives, they were able to adapt and extend this control into their waking lives. In this sense, something that was "virtual" began to have "real" consequences and benefits.

Lucid dreaming occurs during the REM stage of sleep when most vivid dreams occur. However, unlike regular dreaming, lucid dreaming involves a heightened state of awareness and cognitive clarity. In fact, lucid dreaming occurs in the prefrontal cortex (PFC) and temporoparietal junction (TPJ) of the brain, known for self-awareness and perspective-taking, respectively. Normally, REM sleep is characterized by decreased frontal lobe function, leading to reduced critical thinking and self-awareness. Logic is thrown out the window. However, in lucid dreams, partial reactivation of the PFC and connected areas enables reality testing, intentional control, and metacognition (thinking about one's own thoughts).[8] In a similar way, the strong emotional content that is driven by the amygdala in REM sleep is regulated in lucid dreaming through increased PFC-amygdala connectivity. In layman's terms, the highly emotional and illogical structure of normal dreams gives way to less emotion and more logic in lucid dreaming.

This phenomenon is not a new discovery. Tibetan Buddhism, for example, incorporates lucid dreaming into dream yoga, a meditative practice to understand the nature of reality (more on this in the next section). Modern psychology also acknowledges its value in areas such as trauma therapy, problem-solving, and personal growth. Although, just mere years ago, there was no physiological evidence for lucid dreaming, lucid dreamers can now be trained to make prearranged eye sequences that can be electrophysiologically measured to indicate that they are dreaming lucidly. It was the psychologist and dream researcher Stephen LaBerge who proved the existence of lucid dreaming when he created a method in which he made specific eye movements so that his colleagues would know that he was awake during his dreams. This objective confirmation gave lucid dreaming legitimacy in the scientific community, severing its ties from parapsychology and pseudoscience.

At first glance, the idea of "active dreaming" might seem counterproductive to restful sleep. My patients tell me that they want to be less active, spend less energy in sleep, and totally relax. It's their one chance in their busy lives to get away from it all. Why would they want to be aware of their awareness, then? Lucid dreaming can enhance our relationship with sleep in several ways. For individuals who are suffering from recurring nightmares or PTSD, lucid dreaming can serve as a therapeutic tool. By recognizing the dream and taking control of the narrative, the dreamer can transform a frightening scenario into something peaceful or empowering.

Also, the practice of lucid dreaming often involves mindfulness and relaxation techniques, such as reality checks or visualization exercises. These practices can improve overall sleep hygiene and help you fall asleep more easily. And because it provides a means of creating positive or neutral dream experiences, lucid dreaming can make REM sleep, a critical stage for emotional processing, more beneficial.

Lucid dreaming offers a rare opportunity to engage directly with your subconscious mind so you can discover the hidden emotions, unresolved conflicts, or creative insights that might elude you in waking life, where numerous filters and censors abound. In a lucid dream, you can ask questions, confront symbolic fears, or explore environments that reveal deeper truths about your psyche. For instance, encountering a recurring figure in your dreams and interacting with it consciously might shed light on unresolved emotions or patterns. You can ask this figure difficult questions that you may have not had the courage to ask them in real life, such as "Why do you hate me so much?" "I love you, but do you feel the same about me?" "I think we would make great business partners, but what are your qualms about this venture?"

Because the dream world is inherently safe, lucid dreaming can serve as a training ground for facing fears or practicing difficult conversations, as well as boosting confidence and resilience in waking life. For example, if you're contemplating purchasing a sports car but are unsure whether this would be suitable for you, you can take this car on a test drive, as it were, in your dreams. It's a rehearsal of sorts for the real thing, where you can gauge whether it's suitable for your lifestyle. I've found that most of my patients enjoy the novelty of lucid dreaming, but they don't really understand the point of it until they begin to integrate it into their nightly ritual. Once they do, however, they begin to understand how life-altering lucid dreaming can be.

Lucid dreaming can also reduce sleep-related anxiety, which is a major contributor to insomnia. Many people with insomnia fear losing control at night, whether it's the fear of lying awake for hours or of having disturbing dreams. But if you regularly practice lucidity, you develop a sense of confidence and control over your dream world, which can carry over into your waking life. I have found this notion especially powerful with my patients who are deeply anxious about going to sleep. If you know that you can shape your dreams and work with them rather than fight them, nighttime stops feeling so daunting. Instead of dreading sleep, you may even start looking forward to the chance to explore your dreams; you can turn insomnia into an opportunity rather than a struggle.

While lucid dreaming can be exciting and offer insight, it's essential to approach it with balance. Overattachment to achieving lucidity can disrupt sleep, so prioritize relaxation and let lucidity arise naturally. Remember, the goal is not just control but a deeper connection to your inner self, all the while improving your sleep. Initially, as can be expected, most of my patients are concerned about getting the techniques of lucid dreaming just right. They are focused on technique and getting into the dream, but not substance. Once they've cleared this hurdle, though, and can interact with the characters in their dreams, the real excitement begins.

Beyond offering perspective and insight into troubling concerns, lucid dreaming may also enhance certain physical skills—a finding increasingly supported by neuroscience. When you practice movements in a lucid dream, whether it's playing the piano, shooting hoops, or perfecting your golf swing, your brain activates similar neural pathways as when you physically do them in real life. Studies on motor imagery and mental rehearsal show that visualizing an action strengthens the same brain circuits used for actual movement. Because lucid dreaming is a hyper-immersive form of mental practice, it can refine muscle memory, coordination, and even reaction time. The brain doesn't always distinguish between imagined and real experiences, so dream rehearsal can translate into real-world improvements. Athletes, musicians, and even patients have explored this idea to enhance performance. I've occasionally used it with some of my patients, with varying results. Not all of it has been successful, but it is a great starting point and something to try. The key is to engage in detailed, intentional practice within the dream, whether this is feeling the movements, sensing the resistance, or focusing on precision, so your brain encodes it effectively.

As renowned scholar of Buddhism and dream yoga B. Alan Wallace observes, lucid dreaming can "challenge and stretch the limits of identity" and invite you beyond the boundaries of the ego.[9] The true depth of lucid dreaming lies not just in mastering techniques but in the personal journey of self-discovery and transformation it can spark. The practice of lucid dreaming is vast and nuanced—best explored with patience, curiosity, and, if you wish, the guidance of dedicated resources. For those eager to dive deeper, I recommend the work of Stephen LaBerge, whose research laid the foundation for modern lucid-dreaming science, as well as accessible instructions from teachers such as Charlie Morley and Robert Waggoner. Online communities such as r/LucidDreaming on Reddit also offer a variety of resources. Remember, the most profound experiences often come not from following a script but from engaging with your dreams in your own unique way.

Tibetan Dream Yoga

Tibetan Dream Yoga is often seen as the spiritual cousin of lucid dreaming but with a far deeper purpose. Rooted in the Six Yogas of Naropa, this ancient Buddhist practice isn't just about controlling your dreams for fun or creativity—it's about waking up to the true nature of reality. While Western lucid dreaming tends to focus on personal exploration or entertainment, dream yoga uses the dream state as a training ground for enlightenment. Practitioners learn to recognize that both waking life and dreams are illusions—impermanent, shifting, and shaped by perception. If you can wake up inside a dream, the tradition teaches, you can also wake up inside your daily life, seeing through the stories and attachments that usually bind us.

In dream yoga, the goal isn't just to play with the dream world, but to dissolve it, to experience consciousness beyond form, and to prepare for the ultimate transition—death and the bardo, the space between lives. As both a neuroscientist and a student of these teachings, I find it fascinating how dream yoga and lucid dreaming start in the same place—awareness within a dream—but diverge in their aims: One seeks control, the other seeks liberation.

The fundamental goal of Tibetan dream yoga isn't control—it's liberation. In the West, lucidity is often about bending the dream to your will, but in dream yoga, it's about seeing through the illusion altogether. Dream yoga is a spiritual practice that aims to train the mind to recognize all experiences—waking, dreaming, or deep sleep—as part of an illusory, ever-changing reality. By doing this, practitioners develop insight into the nature of existence itself.

Let's say you realize you're dreaming. A lucid dreamer might take off into the sky, summon an old friend, or walk through walls just for the thrill. A dream yoga practitioner, on the other hand, would pause and ask: "What is the dream made of? Who is the 'me' that's dreaming?" Instead of engaging in the dream's story, they work on dissolving the illusion altogether. They're letting go of attachment to the dreamworld just as one learns to let go of attachments in waking life.

Both practices start the same way: You recognize a dream sign. Maybe your hands look strange, or a clock face morphs before your eyes. You realize you're dreaming. While lucid dreamers might stabilize the dream and extend it, dream yoga practitioners may deliberately shift its form, allow themselves to dissolve into light, merge with the void, or recognize that the dream and the dreamer are one. The idea is that by training this awareness in dreams, you can carry it into waking life and, eventually, into the process of dying itself.

Here's where our normal concept of wakefulness is flipped on its head. In the West, we think of being awake as the gold standard of reality: What's real is what we experience with our senses in the daylight hours. But in Buddhist philosophy, waking life is just another kind of dream. It may be a more stable, persistent one, but it's a dream nonetheless. From this perspective, our everyday thoughts, identities, and stories about the world are just fabrications of the mind—not fundamentally different from the illusions we encounter in dreams. Dream yoga is about piercing through this illusion, not just in sleep, but in all of experience. The goal isn't just to be lucid in dreams but to be lucid in life. The intention is to wake up to the deeper truth that the self, as we normally conceive it, is fluid, impermanent, and interconnected with everything.

From this perspective, life itself is seen as a dream, and death is simply a transition into another phase of awareness. Advanced dream yoga practitioners train themselves in lucid dreaming as a preparation for the bardo, the transitional state between death and rebirth. If we remain aware in dreams, the idea is that we can also remain aware after death, navigating the bardo with clarity rather than being swept up in confusion and fear. This is why dream yoga goes beyond the personal thrill of controlling the dream. It's a practice for dying well, for meeting the unknown with awareness rather than unconsciousness. It's about how we move through every moment of existence, waking or dreaming, with presence, insight, and, ultimately, freedom.

So, does this mean lucid dreaming is just shallow entertainment compared to dream yoga? Not necessarily. In fact, lucid dreaming can be a gateway into deeper spiritual practice. If you've ever been lucid in a dream, you already recognize how powerful it feels to wake up inside an illusion. That's the first step. The next step is to use that awareness to question the illusions of waking life. What assumptions do we take for granted? What identities do we cling to? What fears do we avoid? Dream yoga invites us to take lucid dreaming beyond personal curiosity and into the realm of true awakening. It's not about escaping into dreams; it's about waking up to the deeper truth that all of reality is more dreamlike than we think.

Ultimately, what we are going for is *rigpa*, which refers to a state of pure awareness—an unconditioned, ever-present knowing that exists beyond thought. It's often described as the true nature of mind, untouched by distractions, emotions, or the noise of daily life. It is empty of identity yet cognizant. Deep sleep is considered a natural doorway to this state. When we fall asleep, our conceptual mind dissolves, and if we can remain aware during this transition, we can directly experience the luminous clarity of rigpa. This is the reason advanced meditators practice dream yoga and sleep meditation: They are using sleep as a path to awakening rather than just unconscious rest.

Imagine lying in bed, exhausted but restless. Instead of scrolling through your phone or forcing sleep—which you should never do—gently bring your attention to the feeling of simply being. Notice the moment your thoughts begin to blur, that in-between space where wakefulness fades. Normally, you'd black out, but this time, you relax into it, fully present. There's no "you" watching; there's just awareness itself, vast and peaceful. For a moment, it feels like floating in a quiet, infinite space. The next morning, you wake up not just rested, but with a lingering sense of clarity, as if your mind touched something deeper than sleep. That's a glimpse of rigpa.

Dreams as Warnings or Messages of Intuition

Another way to work with your dream is to consider its meaning as if it were warning you, giving you advance notice that something bad is about to happen. Often, these dreams provide life-saving medical insights before any physical symptoms appear to the individual. Dr. Larry Burk, a radiologist and dream researcher, is one of the leading voices on warning dreams, particularly in relation to health. His book, *Dreams That Can Save Your Life,* coauthored with the dream expert Kathleen O'Keefe-Kanavos, presents a fascinating and prescient collection of such real-life accounts where dreams literally saved lives.[10] Burk became interested in this phenomenon after hearing multiple stories of people who dreamed about their illnesses—especially breast cancer—before any medical tests confirmed it. Many of these warning dreams were incredibly vivid and specific, sometimes featuring guides, deceased loved ones, or symbolic imagery pointing directly to the affected body part.

One of the most compelling cases he shares is that of O'Keefe-Kanavos, the coauthor herself. Despite multiple negative mammograms, she kept having recurring dreams in which mysterious figures—sometimes doctors, sometimes monks—told her she had breast cancer. Thankfully and persistently, she pushed for further testing, and a biopsy eventually confirmed the diagnosis. The dream literally saved her life, a "warning" and "saving" dream.

But what is the mechanism by which these dreams work? How can they be situated in this realm of both science and intuition, something that people may dismiss as coincidence or nonsense? Is it a heightened perception that some of us possess, or even a yet-undiscovered cognitive process? Burk suggests that the subconscious mind may pick up on biological changes before they're detectable through medical tests. Whether this is a form of heightened intuition, deep-body awareness, or an unexplained connection between mind and matter, the evidence is compelling enough that he has encouraged doctors to listen when patients report medically relevant dreams. Burk's work challenges the traditional divide between science and intuition, showing that dreams, far from being random nonsense, can sometimes be early warning systems for our health.

So, is there a way we can cultivate these warning dreams, or do they arise spontaneously and involuntarily? With any dream, you can use the process of dream incubation to ensure the dream is aligned with your aim. For example, you can ask for guidance before sleep. Set an intention and ask: "If something is wrong, let my dreams show me." Writing down all your dreams upon waking may also make a warning dream clear, because even seemingly unrelated symbols might reveal patterns over time. Following this thread, paying attention to recurring dreams is helpful. If a dream repeats, it's worth investigating. Finally, trust your intuition; because, ultimately, these types of dreams are very intuitive and grounded in you. Even if tests come back negative, don't ignore a strong gut feeling. Get a second opinion to relieve your anxiety.

Dreams and Astral Projection as a Rehearsal for Death

I never believed in out-of-body experiences—at least, not until one happened to me. The idea of floating outside oneself, of glimpsing another plane of existence, seemed like something out of a film. I wasn't a believer. I outright dismissed such notions. But reality has a way of unraveling what we think we know. My own understanding of life, death, and consciousness shattered the moment my car veered off the highway, metal screeching, glass exploding, the world tilting violently before everything went black.

Blood was trickling down my forehead, warm at first, then cold as everything around me faded. When I opened my eyes—or thought I did—I wasn't in my body. I was above it, a detached spectator, looking at myself, crumpled in the wreckage. I should have felt pain, panic, something. Instead, there was only silence, a strange calm. My mental state was clear. Then I saw her. A woman standing beside me, not in the chaos of the crash but up above it. She reached for me, my body in that wreckage, and without hesitation, my body followed her. I was still observing myself from above, as if I were two bodies, one corporeal and one spiritual. It wasn't like walking. It was like being pulled, weightless, effortless. The world below blurred, distant, like a fading dream. I knew I was somewhere in between, hovering at the edge of something vast and unknown, something larger than anything I could imagine. Some say an out-of-body experience is the brain's way of coping with trauma. Others say you're slipping into another realm, an astral plane beyond the physical world. I don't know what happens. I don't know where I was. I don't know who I was at that moment. But when I finally woke up, gasping for air, pain rushing back into my body, I knew one thing for certain—wherever I had been, it felt just as real as this world, maybe even more so.

In many traditions, the moment we drift beyond the waking world—whether in an out-of-body experience or each night when we go to bed—it's a kind of rehearsal, a dying and a returning. The ancient Egyptians believed the soul slipped free to wander the realms of the dead before dawn called it home again. Tibetan practitioners speak of dream and astral travel as training for the soul's final release. The Tibetan bardo state is often compared to sleep, particularly dreaming, as both involve shifts in consciousness and detachment from physical reality. Sleep is often considered a mini death, a nightly journey through states of consciousness that mirrors the process of dying. As we just discussed with lucid dreaming or Tibetan dream yoga, there is the possibility of becoming aware inside your dream, and if you can do that, you might also be able to navigate the post-death state consciously, increasing the chances of choosing a favorable rebirth or even achieving enlightenment.

From this perspective, every night we go through a mini bardo, a subtle rehearsal for the moment of death. By practicing awareness during sleep, whether through mindfulness, meditation, or dream yoga, we prepare for the ultimate transition. The more conscious we are in sleep, the more prepared we may be when we enter the final bardo of death. Viewed in this way, the connection between sleep and death isn't just metaphorical; it's a spiritual training ground, a nightly opportunity to engage with impermanence, awareness, and the fluid nature of consciousness itself.

In *Death, Intermediate State, and Rebirth in Tibetan Buddhism*, Lati Rinpoche and Jeffrey Hopkins describe the bardo as a time when the mind, freed from the body's constraints, experiences vivid, often hallucinatory visions shaped by past karma.[11] This parallels the dream state in sleep, where mental imprints (or karma in Buddhist terms) generate experiences independent of external stimuli. Just as in deep sleep, where consciousness retracts from our senses, the initial stages of the bardo involve a process of ending in which gross awareness fades, leaving a subtler, dreamlike clarity. Tibetan Buddhist texts suggest that training in recognizing the dream state through lucid dreaming and meditation can prepare one for navigating the bardo, reinforcing the idea that sleep is not just rest but a nightly rehearsal for death and beyond. In other words, we sleep to rehearse the process of dying. To get good at sleep is to get good at dying, because sleep is a nightly rehearsal for the final surrender, an opportunity to practice dissolution with grace. If we can learn to release ourselves into sleep without anxiety, perhaps when the final moment comes, we will meet it not with resistance, but with the same ease we have cultivated each night—floating gently into the unknown.

One of the greatest fears surrounding death is the loss of control—the fear of disappearing, of ceasing to be. Yet every night, we practice letting go like this. And though we may struggle against sleep when anxious or restless, eventually, we succumb. There is a lesson here:

Surrender is not annihilation. Each night, we dissolve. Each morning, we awaken. A dissolution, an awakening. If we begin to see sleep not as a passive act, but as an intentional surrender, we might also start to reshape our relationship with death itself, which can have a profound effect on how we live.

What if, instead of fearing death, we approached it with the same trust we have in sleep? What if we learned to relax into the unknown, to rest in the space between breaths, thoughts, identities? This is the wisdom embedded in the rhythms of our own biology: Death is not an ending but a transition, just as sleep is not an ending but a beginning for the coming day.

Ironically, the more we contemplate death through sleep, the more awake we become in life. Recognizing the temporary nature of our waking existence—just another dream of sorts—allows us to engage more fully, more vividly with life. When we understand that each day is a brief flicker between two vast unknowns, we begin to live differently. Gratitude sharpens. Attachments loosen. We start to see clearly: Every moment is precious because it is fleeting, and that very impermanence is what makes it shine, what makes it matter, what makes it better.

Tonight, when you close your eyes, pay attention. Feel the way the world dissolves, the way you slip between identities, the way consciousness moves through unseen realms. This is not just sleep. This is practice. This is preparation for life and for death. And maybe, this is the beginning of waking up and living a life worth living.

6

TURNING AIR INTO REST WITH BREATHWORK

DEEPER, QUIETER, SLOWER. THIS OPTIMAL WAY OF BREATHING contains within it all that we need to live and sleep well. It's a breath that is free, that is ours, that asks for nothing in return, except what it provides. Breathing is both conscious and unconscious. Absent disease, we'll continue to breathe without noticing it. We can also consciously alter our breathing, which can have significant benefits in every aspect of our lives, especially for insomnia. As the Buddhist monk and peace activist Thich Nhat Hanh observed, the breath is the intersection of the body and mind.[1]

Breathwork refers to the deliberate use of breathing techniques to influence how we feel—physically, mentally, and emotionally. By slowing, deepening, or rhythmically guiding the breath, we can calm the nervous system and restore balance to the body. I'm always surprised that most physicians respond to breathwork as if it were a second-class citizen—not real medicine because it's simple, free, devoid of technology, and can be conducted anywhere. We've all been conditioned to be wary of anything "free" and "simple," because nothing ever is. But the brilliance of breathwork is that it *is* free and carries with it sundry benefits. When you utilize breathwork for sleep, your brain is forced to focus on the breath itself rather than on the chaos that is rummaging around in your mind. When you quiet this noise in your brain, you can reach a state of relaxation sooner and fall asleep quicker.

THE SCIENCE AND SPIRIT OF BREATH

The exchange of inhalation and exhalation is a physiological necessity that sustains life. When you inhale, your diaphragm, a dome-shaped muscle beneath the lungs, contracts and flattens, expanding the chest cavity. Simultaneously, the intercostal muscles between your ribs lift the ribcage, and your lungs expand, creating a vacuum. Air rushes in, rife with oxygen, that is then absorbed into your bloodstream as it travels through the respiratory system. This inhalation process fuels cellular functions and provides the necessary oxygen for energy production.

Conversely, during exhalation, your diaphragm and intercostal muscles relax, allowing your chest cavity to decrease in size. This relaxation increases the pressure within your lungs, forcing air out as a natural response. Your exhale expels carbon dioxide, a metabolic waste product, completing the respiratory cycle.

To maximize the benefits of breathwork, you must also understand the role of the autonomic nervous system (ANS), which governs involuntary bodily functions, including heart rate, digestion, and, crucially, the respiratory system. Divided into the sympathetic and parasympathetic branches, the ANS finely tunes your responses to stress and relaxation. When you are stressed, your sympathetic nervous system kicks in, and your breath quickens and becomes shallow. This response, often known as the fight-or-flight response, prepares your body for immediate action.

Unfortunately, given the extreme stressors in our environments today—everything from overscheduled workdays to unsettled political climates to epidemic chronic illnesses—for most people, the sympathetic branch is in overdrive. When the sympathetic nervous system is overactive, it is more difficult to access the parasympathetic system, which promotes relaxation and calm. This hyperactivity can manifest in many medical conditions, such as hypertension, gastrointestinal disturbances, cardiovascular problems, and other chronic diseases.

The parasympathetic branch of the ANS is what brings us into the rest-and-digest state. Breathwork can play a crucial role in helping us to shift into a parasympathetic mode by slowing the pace of our breathing and allowing the nervous system to enter a state of tranquility. Deep, intentional breaths signal to the body that it's safe out there (whether it may be or not), so we can downshift into relaxation and recovery.

An essential aspect of the nervous system is heart rate variability (HRV), the variation in time between heartbeats. Breathwork, particularly techniques emphasizing diaphragmatic breathing and controlled inhalation and exhalation, enhance HRV, which, in turn, fosters resilience and adaptability. This embodied connection to the heart is what makes breathwork a powerful bridge between body, mind, and spirit—a theme echoed in both scientific research and ancient wisdom traditions.

As founder of Mindfulness-Based Stress Reduction Jon Kabat-Zinn suggests, "Recognize that in a very real way, the body is doing the breathing, not you. It is more like you are being breathed than that it is you, whoever you think you are, who is doing the breathing."[2] His instruction reflects a key principle of mindfulness and nonduality: a way of experiencing reality in which the usual split between "self" and "world," "mind" and "body," or "observer" and "experience" begins to dissolve. Rather than seeing ourselves as separate from what's happening, awareness recognizes that we are part of the happening itself. He invites us to recognize that many fundamental aspects of our existence are happening beyond our deliberate control. In this sense, we are being breathed and our conscious selves are more like witnesses to the breathing. Rather than forcing, analyzing, or resisting life, we can observe and allow it to unfold naturally, just like breathing and sleeping.

Similarly, Pema Chödrön, a leading figure in the Shambhala Buddhist tradition, uses the compassion practice of *tonglen*, where one breathes in the suffering of themselves or others, and breathes out relief, kindness, or whatever is most needed.[3] But why would we breathe in pain? Why relish in something that's uncomfortable? It's not about taking on more; it's about transforming our relationship to discomfort. In the context of sleep, tonglen can be grounding. When anxiety or restlessness keeps us up, we try breathing in that tight, hot feeling with the intention, "I'm not the only one feeling this tonight." Then we breathe out calm, sending it to ourselves and anyone else struggling, too. It turns breath into a channel for compassion, not just for us, but for the whole sleepless world. It's time, then, that we use our body and breath to heal, which is the philosophy behind integrative medicine and these breathing techniques.

INTEGRATING BREATHWORK INTO A NIGHTTIME ROUTINE

Breathing techniques work. However, practice and persistence are key. You cannot just do them once and have immediate success. Yes, you may see immediate benefits, but for real progress, you'll want to make these breathing techniques a well-ingrained, natural extension of your daily life. The best way to do that is by establishing a consistent nighttime routine, pairing relaxing breathwork with other calming rituals.

Here are some ways to begin:

- *Create a relaxing environment.* Dim the lights, put your phone on Do Not Disturb, and maybe even light a candle or use an essential oil diffuser with lavender or chamomile.
- *Find a comfortable spot to practice.* You can conduct breathwork lying in a bed, sitting on a cushion, or lying on the floor with a blanket. The key is to feel supported and at ease.
- *Set a timer.* Start with just five to ten minutes. This keeps it approachable and ensures you're not checking the clock during your practice.
- *Use guided audio practices.* There are many online sources, including meditation apps, that will guide you through some of these practices until they become second nature to you.
- *Combine breathwork with other routines.* Pair it with journaling, a warm bath, or reading a relaxing book. It doesn't have to be a standalone activity.
- *Do it at the same time each day.* Whether that's after brushing your teeth or just before turning off the lights, do a breathing practice, even if it's just for a minute or two.

Breathwork isn't just about falling asleep faster. It's also about creating a space to decompress and let go of the day. In our busy, overstimulated world, taking even a few minutes to focus on your breath can feel like a small act of rebellion. It's a way of saying, "I deserve to rest." And in that pause, in that quiet calm of space, you will start to remember what it feels like to simply be. Not productive. Not performing. Not negotiating. Just human. And, sometimes, that's all it takes to begin to sleep better and heal.

BREATHWORK PRACTICES FOR IMPROVING SLEEP

The following practices (with the exception of the final two practices) will help you calm an overactive nervous system and establish the physiological conditions to welcome sleep more easily.

The 4-7-8 Breath

Also known as the relaxing breath, the 4-7-8 breath induces relaxation almost immediately and can be done anywhere, anytime. Developed by Dr. Andrew Weil, this breathing method is ideal for anyone who experiences insomnia related to anxiety. It can also be useful in any stressful situation when you're stressed, frustrated, and irritable.

1. Place the tip of your tongue just behind your upper front teeth and keep it there for the remainder of the exercise.
2. Exhale through your mouth, making a *whoosh* sound.
3. Close your mouth and inhale quietly through your nose to a mental count of four.
4. Hold your breath for seven seconds.
5. Exhale completely through your mouth, making a *whoosh* sound to a count of eight seconds. This would be considered one breath.
6. Inhale again and repeat the cycle three more times for a total of four breaths.

It's vital to remember to inhale through your nose and exhale through your mouth. The amount of time spent on each phase is not as important as the ratio—make sure your exhale is twice as long as your inhale. With time, this technique will become so natural that you'll unconsciously use it during both stressful situations and when attempting to initiate and maintain sleep. If I could choose only one breathing technique, this would be the one.

Paced Nostril Breathing

Also known as alternate nasal breathing, or *nadi shodhana*, paced nostril breathing is like hitting the brain's dimmer switch. It slows your breath, balances your nervous system, and according to EEG studies, can increase calming alpha and theta brain waves—the very rhythms of calm and transition. Alpha waves (8–12 Hz) are the gentle, wakeful rhythms linked with relaxed focus and quiet alertness, while theta waves (4–8 Hz) emerge in meditation, drowsiness, and the borderlands of sleep. Together, these slower oscillations mirror the shift from doing to being that breathing practice invites.[4] It's a simple, portable way to prepare your mind for rest or focus, and it works fast. It's my second go-to breath technique after the 4-7-8 technique.

1. Find a comfortable seat. Sit upright, relaxed but alert; cross-legged or in a chair is fine. Let your shoulders drop.
2. Using your right hand close off your right nostril with your thumb.
3. Inhale slowly through your left nostril (about four to five seconds).
4. Close the left nostril with your ring finger, then release the right nostril.
5. Exhale slowly through your right nostril (about four to five seconds).
6. Inhale through your right nostril (same pace), then close it again with your thumb.
7. Exhale through your left nostril.

That's one full cycle. Repeat for five to ten rounds, or about five minutes.

Abdominal Breathing

Abdominal breathing, also called diaphragmatic breathing, is a simple but powerful technique to help you breathe more efficiently and feel more relaxed. Unlike shallow chest breathing, which can make you feel tense or short of breath, abdominal breathing engages your diaphragm, the large muscle beneath your lungs, to draw in deeper, more oxygen-rich breaths. This kind of breathing can lower stress, improve focus, and even help with sleep. In addition, it's a great tool for managing anxiety or calming your nervous system in moments of high tension.

1. Find a comfortable spot. Sit or lie down in a relaxed position. If you're sitting, keep your back straight but not stiff.
2. Put one hand on your chest and the other on your abdomen, just below your ribs. This helps you feel the movement of your breath.
3. Take a slow, deep breath in through your nose. Let the air fill your abdomen, allowing your belly to rise while keeping your chest relatively still.
4. Purse your lips slightly and exhale slowly out your mouth, feeling your belly fall as you release the air.
5. Repeat the steps, continuing for a few minutes, focusing on the rhythm of your breath. If your mind wanders, gently bring your attention back to your breathing.

Try practicing this for a few minutes each day, especially before bed or during stressful times.

Meditative Breathing

Meditative breathing is a simple practice that helps quiet your mind, reduce stress, and bring a sense of calm. It's all about focusing on your breath and being present in the moment. Unlike regular breathing, meditative breathing is intentional—you are fully aware of each inhale and exhale, which can slow racing thoughts and ease anxiety. It's often used in meditation, but you don't need to sit cross-legged for hours to benefit from it. Just a few minutes can help you feel more centered and relaxed.

1. Find a quiet space. Sit or lie down in a comfortable position. If you're sitting, keep your back straight but relaxed.
2. Close your eyes. This helps minimize distractions, but if you're more comfortable with your eyes open, just soften your gaze.
3. Take a deep breath in through your nose. Slowly inhale, filling your lungs completely. Feel the air expand your chest and belly.
4. Exhale gently through your mouth or nose. As you exhale, become aware of any bodily tension, and let it go.
5. Continue breathing in a slow, steady pattern. You can count (like inhaling for four seconds and exhaling for six) or simply notice the natural flow of your breath.
6. Bring your mind back to your breath when it wanders. If thoughts pop up (and they will), don't worry. Just gently guide your focus back to your breath.

Continue to do this breathing technique for five to ten minutes until you feel sleepy.

Breathwork Visualization

Focusing on the many characteristics of your breathing, such as rhythm, will facilitate the onset of your sleep. By picturing the breath as something you can see, feel, or even hear within you, you begin to bridge imagination and body awareness. Focusing on the many characteristics of your breathing—its rhythm, texture, and flow—gently draws your attention inward and helps quiet the mind, facilitating the onset of sleep.

1. Lie down in bed and focus on relaxation.
2. Feel the bed supporting you as you exhale.
3. As you become more relaxed, focus on your exhales and notice how you feel. Do you feel as if you're sinking into the bed? Do you feel like things are slowing down? Do you feel heavier or more solid?
4. Shift your attention to both the inhale and exhale. Visualize the colors, shapes, or other images that come to you as you observe the quality of your breath. Slip into the experience and let yourself drift into your imagination.

Repeat these steps until you feel drowsy and fall asleep.

Counting While Breathing

While counting sheep has long been a popular folk technique for falling asleep, contemporary research suggests it may not offer much benefit and may even delay sleep onset in some cases. For example, studies have found that imagining a calming scene helped people fall asleep approximately twenty minutes faster than counting sheep, which turned out to be either no better than doing nothing or slightly worse.[5] However, many of my patients have more luck with counting sheep's close cousin, counting while breathing.

1. Lie down in bed. Exhale calmly and slowly.
2. Feel the bed supporting you.
3. Count slowly from one to ten and then back from ten to one, letting each number flow with the length of your exhale. Begin counting as the breath starts to leave the body, and let the number fade as the exhale softens to its end.

Repeat this sequence until you fall asleep.

The Humming Bee Breath

The humming bee breath, also known as *bhramari pranayama,* is a breathing technique that involves making a deep, steady humming sound while exhaling. This breath is often practiced as a form of meditation to calm the mind, reduce stress, promote relaxation, and improve insomnia. It can also be used as a tool to help improve focus and concentration. Numerous studies have shown that this type of breathing is associated with relaxation, improved cognition and memory, and reduced anxiety.[6] Heart rate and blood pressure may also decrease with this breathing technique.

1. Find a comfortable position: Sit comfortably with your spine straight, either on the floor or in a chair. You can also practice lying down if that's more comfortable for you.
2. Close your eyes and take a few deep breaths. Begin to relax your body and mind.
3. Place your thumbs on your ears. Place your index fingers just above your eyebrows, and the rest of your fingers lightly over your eyes. Alternatively, you can simply place your index fingers on your ears without covering your eyes.
4. Take a slow, deep breath in through your nose, filling your lungs completely.
5. As you exhale, gently press your fingers against your ears to partially close them, and then make a steady humming sound, like the buzzing of a bee. The sound should be deep and resonant.
6. Concentrate on the vibration and sound of the humming as you exhale. Feel the vibrations reverberating throughout your head and body.
7. Continue to inhale deeply through your nose and exhale with the humming sound for several rounds, maintaining a slow and steady pace.

After completing the practice, take a moment to notice how you feel. Notice any changes in your body, breath, or state of mind.

The Bellows Breath

The bellows breath is a yogic breathing technique, also known as *bhastrika pranayama*. It involves rapid inhalations and exhalations through the nose to clear the mind. It's so named because it resembles a bellows blasting air onto coals of a fire. Imaging of the brain via functional magnetic resonance imaging (fMRI) during such a technique reveals reduced functional connectivity in certain regions of the brain, which, as a result, causes decreased anxiety. This reduced anxiety can improve insomnia. However, this breath is also quite stimulating, so it is best practiced in the morning or at least a few hours before you go to bed.

1. Find a comfortable position. Sit with your spine straight, either on the floor or in a chair. You can also practice lying down if that's more comfortable for you.
2. Relax. Close your eyes and take a few deep breaths to relax your body and mind.
3. Begin rapidly breathing. Inhale and exhale rapidly and forcefully through your nose. The breaths should be short and quick, like the pumping action of a bellows. The movement should come from your diaphragm, so your abdomen should rise and fall with each breath.
4. Keep the rhythm steady and consistent, aiming for around thirty breaths per minute or whatever pace feels comfortable for you. It's essential to maintain control and not overexert yourself.
5. Concentrate on the sensation of the breath moving in and out of the nostrils. You can also visualize the breath energizing your body with each inhalation and releasing tension with each exhalation.

6. Start with a short session of one to two minutes and gradually increase the duration as you become more comfortable with the technique.
7. After your practice session, return to normal breathing and take a few moments to notice how you feel. Reflect on any changes in your body, breath, or state of mind.

It's essential to practice bellows breathing mindfully and to listen to your body. If you feel dizzy, lightheaded, or uncomfortable at any point, stop the practice and return to normal breathing. As with any breathing technique, consistency and patience are key to experiencing its benefits over time.

7

SHADOW WORK AND EMOTIONAL HEALING

My family and I left Iran in 1979 during the hostage crisis, when headlines painted Iranians as villains and fear ran high. My grandfather worked for the shah of Iran, holding a respected position that, before the Islamic Revolution, gave our family both pride and a sense of security. The shah believed in the vision of a modern, progressive Iran—one where education, culture, and diplomacy flourished. But when the tides shifted during the revolution, everything changed almost overnight. Those who had served the shah or were associated with the old regime became targets. Whispers turned to threats, and our family, once rooted in the fabric of Tehran's professional class, was suddenly under siege. Fear crept into our home. We could no longer speak freely, and my grandfather's legacy, once a badge of honor, became a source of extreme danger.

We fled Iran not as travelers but as exiles, leaving behind a life that had been carefully built over generations. After a brief stay in the Netherlands, we arrived in the United States. I was just a kid, but I knew enough to stay quiet about where I came from. On the first day of school in Southern California, I remember shrinking a little when someone asked me where I was from. I mumbled something vague and changed the subject. I didn't want to be the target of side-eyes or the butt of another hostage joke, so I started editing myself. I softened my name and Americanized the pronunciation, avoided speaking Farsi in public, and did everything I could to not seem "Iranian." What I didn't realize was that I wasn't just trying to fit in: I was splitting off a part of myself—a part I hid away and would later come to know as my shadow.

WHO IS THIS STRANGER WITHIN?

The shadow is our double-walker, or inner *doppelgänger,* as it is known in German. In literature, they often represent duality, hidden aspects of identity, or moral conflicts that we may not recognize in ourselves. Your shadow is the parts of your personality that you have disowned. These parts feel "shady," like a companion following us like a shadow, always there, but somehow untouchable. As children, we learn to identify with what's acceptable and shun what is not. This creates a split in our psyche—a sense of holding something back, not revealing our true selves. Carl Jung called the shadow the part of us that we don't want to be part of us. We repress it and often project our shame onto others.

But what happens to it? Where does it go, this aspect of us that Jung named the shadow? Repressed, it becomes more independent, always lurking, trying to find expression. The more we fight it, the stronger it becomes. It derives its power from the energy that we use to suppress it, a coil that is wound so tightly that it'll spring when we least expect it. Often, we project our shadow parts—the traits that our shadow holds—onto others, both those we love as well as strangers or foreigners. This seems like a perfect solution because we have thrown out the "trash," as it were, and we can temporarily feel free of it by acknowledging it in others. But the shadow lies within, ready to pounce at a moment's notice, causing us anxiety, hatred, and insomnia. So how to best resolve this entanglement? It is by recognizing the shadow, acknowledging that it resides with us, and integrating it that we can finally be honest and happy with ourselves and others whom we have scapegoated. We have created anxiety and fear around a shadow that is just us—us in a form that we don't recognize yet.

The enduring intrigue surrounding the shadow lies in its ability to evoke questions about identity, reality, and the nature of the self. We'd like to think these double-walkers are greedy, foreigners, scumbags, who want nothing else but to take our enjoyment away from us and rob us from ourselves. To the shadow, you may say: "Hey, asshole, what are you doing following me?" "Get away from me; you look disheveled, you smell!" "So, now, you're following me, trying to invade my home, marry my partner, eat my food, and sleep in my bed? Eh? I won't allow it! I'll sooner kill you, you pathetic thief, than let you destroy the life that I've built so well! I'm a respected member of this society, and damn you if you want to destroy my reputation alongside yours!" We tell ourselves that we cannot allow the doppelgänger, the foreigner, the shadow, to become part of our lives; because then, who are we, who do we become? But the irony of this type of thinking is that the doppelgänger is us. It is the foreigner within us, that part of ourselves we refuse to nurture, which has now come to exact revenge. If only we had communicated with it, understood its needs, recognized that it only wanted to be heard, just like we do, then we wouldn't be so anxious, so afraid, so envious of its radical indifference.

The French psychoanalyst Julia Kristeva explores this idea that the "foreigner" isn't just an external outsider; it's something within us, an unfamiliar part of our own psyche that we often repress.[1] This is akin to Carl Jung's concept of the shadow, which represents the hidden, unacknowledged aspects of ourselves—the impulses, desires, and fears we push into the unconscious. Both Kristeva and Jung suggest that what we reject or fear in others is often a reflection of what we haven't accepted in ourselves. The Kristevan stranger and the Jungian shadow are unsettling because they reveal that we are not as solid and self-contained as we'd like to believe. There's something within us that resists full integration, something foreign that lingers at the edges of our identity.

This idea has profound implications for anxiety, especially the kind that surfaces around sleep. Insomnia and bedtime anxiety often stem from a fear of losing control, of drifting into the unknown where the unconscious takes over. But what if part of our restlessness comes from resisting the stranger within? What if sleep is terrifying precisely because it dissolves the boundaries of the self, forcing us to confront aspects of our psyche we'd rather avoid? Instead of treating nighttime anxiety as something to suppress or fight, maybe the Kristevan approach would be to welcome it as a sign that something in us wants to be recognized. Just like Jung encouraged dialogue with the shadow, Kristeva's stranger invites us to make peace with the unfamiliar, both inside and outside ourselves. Perhaps sleep itself is a kind of surrender to this inner foreigner, an acceptance of the strangeness within all of us.

Lessons from Dr. Jekyll and Mr. Hyde

The Strange Case of Dr. Jekyll and Mr. Hyde, Robert Louis Stevenson's dark tale of duality, provides us with a literary exploration of this concept of a shadow.[2] By examining the trustworthy and respected Dr. Jekyll's transformation into the monstrous Hyde, who surreptitiously kills people in the quiet hours of the night, we can see the dangers of neglecting the shadow and learn how integrating it is essential for our emotional well-being, including our relationship with sleep.

Dr. Jekyll embodies the socially accepted persona: a man of propriety and moral standing, a physician. This persona, however, is limiting. He can't do anything he'd like because he must represent to the world that he is a man in good standing. His alter ego, Mr. Hyde, is the unrestrained embodiment of his suppressed desires and darker impulses. Mr. Hyde has free rein to do whatever he'd like because he has no persona. He has no identity to project to the world, so he can be as disruptive as he'd like. He can create chaos like no other. Hyde emerges not because Jekyll is inherently evil (though that is sometimes how this story is taught), but because he represses parts of himself that he deems unacceptable to himself and others.

Jung argued that ignoring the shadow causes psychological imbalance, as the repressed aspect of the self requires expression, and it will seek it in increasingly destructive ways if it finds no outlet. This repressed part, this foreigner, this shadow, hasn't been acknowledged. It wants to be heard because it has something important to say. But we don't allow it to speak because we are fearful of what it has to say about us, about the way it can destroy our lives, because we've been living a life that is so good, but also so very inauthentic. But the more we fail to listen to the shadow, the more power it exerts over us. Through Jekyll's inability to control Hyde once he is unleashed, Stevenson warns us of the misfortune that can occur when we fail to acknowledge and integrate our shadow selves. Hyde's nocturnal wanderings and indulgences—his kills—serve as a metaphor for how suppressed emotions, longings, and unresolved inner conflicts will surface when we let our guard down, often at night.

Jung observed that the shadow often reveals itself in dreams, which act as a bridge to the unconscious. In Stevenson's novella, the transformations where Jekyll becomes Hyde frequently occur at night, highlighting how the darkness and solitude of night provide fertile ground for repressed emotions to emerge. Similarly, when we sleep, our defenses lower, allowing the shadow to manifest in dreams or even in the form of insomnia, because unresolved inner conflicts disrupt our rest.

Dreams of being chased, guilt-ridden, or out of control can symbolize the shadow's attempt to communicate with us. These themes are Jung's way of reminding us that ignoring the shadow, whether through suppression or avoidance, does not make it disappear; instead, it often causes restlessness and anxiety that causes disturbed sleep.

The place to start is to initiate dialogue with the shadow. Let it tell you about yourself when the light is dim, when darkness abounds, where we can lurk in the shadows with it, just for a bit, in the hope that we can allow it a glimpse of a light—perhaps less at first, but more eventually, as we grow more comfortable with its presence.

The Strange Case of Dr. Jekyll and Mr. Hyde teaches us that facing and integrating the shadow is essential for a balanced psyche and restful sleep. Shadow work, the process of bringing hidden parts of ourselves into conscious awareness, can have profound implications for mental health and sleep. Suppressing aspects of ourselves creates internal conflict, so acknowledging inner tensions reduces stress, which can lead to better sleep. Similarly, integrating our shadows (there is usually more than one) brings wholeness and a sense of peace when the unconscious mind is allowed to rest rather than wrestle with denial. And, perhaps most importantly, the guilt and shame that accompany shadow repression often feed sleepless nights. Accepting and working through these emotions can break this cycle, fostering a healthier relationship with rest and sleep.

Stevenson's novella reminds us that the shadow is not inherently evil; it's simply the unacknowledged part of ourselves. Hyde's downfall is not his existence but rather Jekyll's refusal to integrate him into a balanced whole. As Jung teaches us, when we face the dark corners of our minds, we not only find inner peace but also improve the quality of our sleep and overall well-being. The alchemy of turning shadow into light, of integrating the shadow into our persona—much like Jekyll's unfulfilled quest—requires courage and honesty. Shadow work is how we'll proceed.

SHADOW WORK AND SLEEP

When we ponder what keeps us up at night, we often look toward obvious culprits: caffeine, stress, blue light from our phones, the usual suspects. But for some, the problem runs deeper, tethered to unresolved fears and buried conflicts lurking beneath the surface of consciousness. These hidden factors, our "shadow selves," can be profound disruptors of restorative sleep. Shadow work offers a powerful framework for exploring and addressing these hidden elements.

To do shadow work means you will begin to think about the parts of you that have been shunned and unconsciously repressed; those shadows that have been concealed by your persona, the mask that you wear daily. These are the shadows that you will be confronting and befriending. They may be at the root of your pernicious insomnia and poor sleep, especially if you are not getting any relief from treatments such as hypnotics or CBT-I. As Jung suggests, if we are able to see our own shadow and can bear knowing about it, then a small part of the problem has already been solved: We have at least brought up the personal unconscious. Being able to validate one's feelings to see aspects of our personality in a different light is enough for some people to improve or even resolve their insomnia.

At its core, shadow work involves bringing unconscious aspects of ourselves—our shadows—into conscious awareness. The shadow includes traits, emotions, and experiences that we suppress or reject, often because they conflict with our self-image or societal expectations. While this repression can help us navigate daily life, it comes at a cost: The shadow doesn't disappear. Instead, it lurks in the background and simmers in the unconscious, manifesting in subtle and not-so-subtle ways, including anxiety, nightmares, and sleeplessness.

Think of the shadow as a backpack of unacknowledged baggage we carry. If the backpack is too full, it weighs us down, even if we don't consciously feel its weight. Shadow work helps us unpack that load.

Unresolved fears and conflicts often emerge at night, when the distractions of the day fade and our minds are left to wander. These can take many forms. Unaddressed fears may cause looping thoughts that prevent us from falling asleep. Repressed emotions can seep into dream content, disrupting our sleep architecture. Emotional suppression often manifests as physical tension, which can make it difficult to relax into sleep.

Shadow work often gets framed as mysterious or intimidating, but at its heart, it's simply about understanding ourselves more fully. When we repress certain emotions or traits, they don't just vanish. Instead, they linger in the unconscious, subtly influencing our thoughts, behaviors, and relationships. Over time, this disconnection from parts of ourselves can lead to anxiety, irritability, and feelings of being "stuck," all of which cause or contribute to insomnia. Shadow work helps to bridge this gap.

Unresolved shadow elements often show up as strong emotional reactions, or "triggers." For instance, if you find yourself deeply annoyed when someone is boastful, it may reflect a part of you that craves recognition but has been suppressed. If you are full of judgment when someone is shy, this may reflect an intolerance of your own internal sense of caution or doubt. By acknowledging and working with this aspect, you reduce the emotional charge and power behind it. As a result, you feel calmer and more in control, which fosters emotional resilience.

Our unresolved shadows often spill into our relationships, leading to misunderstandings or conflict. For example, if you've suppressed your need for boundaries, you might harbor resentment when others cross them, even if you never articulated them. Shadow work helps you recognize these patterns and communicate more authentically and effectively. As a result, you may experience stronger, more fulfilling relationships with yourself and others.

Emotional suppression doesn't just affect your mind; it also impacts your body. Repressed feelings can create physical tension, which interferes with your ability to relax and fall asleep. Through shadow work, you can release these emotions, leading to a deeper state of relaxation, as well as easier sleep onset and fewer disruptions throughout the night.

Shadow work involves confronting parts of yourself you might prefer to ignore—jealousy, anger, fear—and it's important to do so with curiosity, kindness, and patience. This isn't quick or easy work. Bringing unconscious material into the light takes persistence, honesty, and often support. There are many techniques and resources available, from journaling and guided exercises to workshops and therapy. You may find it helpful to have the support of a therapist, especially when starting out. Ultimately, shadow work is a journey, not a destination—one that unfolds over time and can lead to profound healing. Let me share with you how this process went for one of my patients.

Safran's Story

Safran was a thirty-five-year-old marketing professional known for her strong work ethic and attention to detail. She was always the first to arrive and the last to leave, priding herself on being the go-to problem solver. But this dedication came at a cost: late nights, missed weekends, and growing frustration when others didn't meet her high standards. I first saw Safran for insomnia, but it quickly became clear her sleeplessness was tied to deeper issues. She found herself snapping at her team and feeling resentful when they didn't show the same level of commitment.

After a heated argument with a colleague, she began to wonder why she felt so overwhelmed and dissatisfied. These issues soon began to affect her sleep. Previously, Safran slept well and woke refreshed. But after her argument at work, she started waking up in the middle of the night, unable to stop ruminating about her job and her own high expectations. Despite her professional success, Safran told me she felt empty. She shared feelings of vulnerability, imperfection, and even anger or envy toward colleagues who set boundaries or prioritized their personal lives. She realized she denied herself the right to make mistakes or take breaks and projected her frustration onto others who did. Beneath her perfectionism, she discovered a fear of not being "enough" that she tried to mask by always going above and beyond.

I suspected her struggle was really about a conflict between her identity as a high-achieving perfectionist and the parts of herself she tried to hide—her shadow—so we began to explore this together. Shadow work became especially helpful for Safran. She started by noticing her emotional triggers—her frustration with colleagues, her urge to overwork, and the emptiness she felt. When she felt anger toward a coworker who left work on time, she asked herself, "Why does this bother me so much? What might this be saying about me?" Like many, Safran's shadow had roots in childhood. As the only girl among three brothers, her worth was tied to achievement.

As Safran began to acknowledge her shadow, she learned to embrace her imperfections and allowed herself to make small mistakes without spiraling into guilt. She started setting boundaries, which helped reduce resentment toward others. Eventually, she began working with a therapist familiar with Jungian concepts to continue this process of acknowledging and integrating her shadow.

WORKING WITH SHAME

Out of all traits that we are inclined to hide, shame is perhaps the most universal. We push away whatever makes us feel as though we are defective, trash, no good. As the psycho-spiritual teacher Robert Augustus Masters rightly notes, "Shame infiltrates us in an instant, bringing our defenses down. We're then like a snail stripped of its shell—naked, soft, and suddenly, so, so vulnerable."[3] Most of us will do anything to avoid this feeling, including retreating into extreme behaviors such as aggression, emotional disconnection, and narcissism. Shame is much more insidious, much more dangerous than guilt. Guilt says, *I did something bad.* Shame whispers, *I am bad.* It buries itself deep, deeper than we'd like, shaping the way we see ourselves and the world around us. If left unchecked, shame becomes a powerful force in our shadow and can infiltrate our sleep, leaving us restless and anxious at night.

We don't like to talk about shame. Instead, we cover it up; we mask it with perfectionism, defensiveness, or even anger. But because it's part of our shadow, it doesn't disappear just because we ignore it. It festers in the background, showing up in ways that we don't expect: self-doubt, imposter syndrome, fear of exposure. It keeps us from speaking up, from taking risks, from living fully. And for many, it keeps us from sleeping, from getting rest. When shame is buried in the shadow, it creates an internal battle: One part of us wants to move forward, indeed desires it like nothing else, while the other drags us back, afraid of judgment, rejection, or exposure. So how do we work through it? While many people explore these exercises on their own, this is deep psychological terrain, and professional guidance can be invaluable. A trained therapist or counselor can help ensure that the process remains constructive and integrated rather than overwhelming.

Like all shadow work, the first step is to identify it. Shame has a script that is deceptive, not accurate. It tells us things about ourselves that feel absolute, but they aren't the truth; they're stories we've absorbed through the years. It produces a lot of evidence to bolster its story, but it ignores any evidence you share to counter it. Start by noticing where shame comes up for you: What parts of yourself do you try to hide from others? Why? When did you first feel it was necessary to hide these things? Write down the words that come up and the images that are conjured by those experiences. Sometimes they sound like, "I'm not good enough, never was." "I'll always fail." "If people knew the real me, they wouldn't stay because I'm no good, I'm trash." Recognizing these messages is the first step in dismantling them.

Next, find the origin of the shame, which is often learned. Somewhere, sometime, along the way, you were told—directly or indirectly—that something about you was unacceptable. At school, they may have called you ugly, smelly, shrimpy, hairy, and a host of other bad depictions; you've carried these traits with you, however inaccurate or exaggerated, through childhood and into adulthood. You may intellectually understand that that's not you, but somewhere deep inside, the beliefs fester and percolate; and on some level, you believe those exaggerated ideas, and it makes you ashamed, disgusted. Ask yourself: "When was the first time I felt ashamed of this part of myself?" "Who made me feel this way? A parent? A teacher? Peers? Society?" "Was this really *my* belief, or did I inherit it?" Often, we carry shame that doesn't belong to us, but we've been indoctrinated to believe it, especially when this shame has been tethered to us in our formative years. Recognizing its source helps loosen shame's grip and establish a perspective that we may not have had at the time of the occurrence.

Many of our deepest shames started when we were children, at a time when we didn't have the tools to process them. Shadow work invites us to reconnect with that child, the part of us still holding on to those wounds, the part of us that's still crying in the bathroom long after the incident, erroneously believing that we are not that good, never were that good, cannot be that good. Close your eyes and imagine your younger self, the version of you who first felt that shame.

What do they look like? How do they feel? Instead of judging them, try compassion. Speak to them as you would a scared child. "I see you. You didn't deserve to feel that way. You were just trying your best. You did nothing wrong. It's the others who should be ashamed because they projected their ugliness, their shame, onto you." This isn't about erasing the past; rather, it's about rewriting the way we carry it.

Expressing what has been suppressed is a powerful tool and one way to out shame, because shame thrives in secrecy. The more we hide shame, like all shadow attributes, the stronger it becomes. One of the most effective ways to weaken shame's hold is through expression. Write a letter to shame. Let it speak, then respond with understanding. More importantly, give a voice to shame and speak it aloud. Even if it's just to yourself in a mirror, putting shame into words takes away its power, its glory.

Finally, once you have exposed and accepted shame as a part of you, you can transform its power into strength. In fact, all the parts of yourself that you hide may just be the key to your greatest powers. What if the thing you're ashamed of is your gift, the gift that sets you apart from others and makes you the extraordinary person you are? Relish this fact. The child who was too sensitive becomes the adult who is deeply empathetic. The person who felt unworthy learns to value themself and inspires others to do the same. The one who was silenced finds their voice and finally uses it to write a beautiful novel or produce and star in a film that touches millions. The one who didn't think they were creative learns to craft and finds community and acceptance among other craftspeople. Shame loses its grip when we see that our wounds shape us and don't define us. We see that they actually reflect something wonderful about us. There's nothing shameful about being human. And when we stop running from the parts of ourselves that we once feared and found shameful or disgusting, we find something unexpected on the other side: freedom. And sleep.

JOURNALING PROMPTS AND EXERCISES

Shadow work is a deeply personal journey, and journaling serves as one of its most accessible and effective tools. Writing allows you to explore the unconscious in a way that is both safe and private, turning abstract emotions and hidden fears into tangible words on a page. Journaling bridges the gap between conscious awareness and the unconscious mind. By giving yourself permission to write freely, you bypass the inner critic and create space for suppressed thoughts, emotions, and patterns to surface. The act of writing also promotes reflection, helping you make connections that might otherwise remain obscured. Journaling also offers you a concrete record of your shadow work journey. Over time, it becomes a mirror reflecting your growth and the patterns you've unraveled, making it easier to see progress and integrate insights into your life.

Below are some journaling prompts and exercises designed to help you uncover, process, and integrate your shadow elements. Before diving into the exercises, it's important to set the stage for this work. Patients often feel it's helpful to journal before going to bed—it seems to get some of the negative thoughts out of their head, leaving room for sleep to enter. Find a comfortable, distraction-free environment where you can focus. Begin each session by grounding yourself. Take a few deep breaths and remind yourself that shadow work is a process of self-discovery, not self-judgment. Resist the urge to edit or censor your thoughts. Let your words flow and allow your unconscious to speak freely, even if they don't make immediate sense.

- *Noticing reactivity and triggers.* Reactivity—those moments when you feel triggered, irritated, or defensive—is often a sign of shadow material surfacing. Recognizing these reactions is the first step toward working with your shadow.

  What recent event or interaction left you feeling overly reactive, irritated, or defensive?

Why might this have bothered you so deeply?

What triggered you today, and what might it reveal about your shadow?

How did you respond in the moment, and how might you respond differently next time?

- *Spotting projection.* Projection happens when we attribute our own unwanted qualities to others. By noticing these projections, we can begin to reclaim and integrate these parts of ourselves.

  When have you caught yourself judging someone harshly? Could this trait exist in you, too?

  What qualities do you find intolerable in others? Hint: look for qualities you think you don't have (e.g., short temper, rigidity, overly talkative).

  What qualities do you admire in others but feel are missing or underdeveloped in yourself (e.g., poise, eloquence, kindness)?

- *Facing your fears.* Our deepest fears often hide in the shadow. Bringing them into the light can be uncomfortable but ultimately freeing.

  What are you most afraid of people knowing about you? Why does this feel so threatening?

  What fear or worry keeps resurfacing in your life, disturbing your sleep? What might it be trying to teach you?

- *Revisiting the past.* The shadow often forms around unprocessed memories or childhood wounds. Exploring these can reveal valuable insights.

  Is there a memory or experience you avoid thinking about? Why do you shy away from it?

  Who or what hurt you in the past? How do you carry that pain today?

- *Embracing repressed desires.* The shadow isn't just about pain—it also contains hidden wishes and potential. Exploring these can lead to growth and fulfillment.

What do you secretly wish you could do but don't allow yourself to pursue? Why do you hold yourself back?

If you could live without fear of judgment, how would your life look different?

- *Learning from dreams and symbols.* Dreams often reveal shadow elements through recurring themes and symbolic characters. Paying attention to these can help you understand and integrate your shadow.

  What recurring themes or images appear in your dreams? How might these connect to your waking life?

  If you were to meet your shadow as a person, what would they look like, and what would they say to you?

  What is your unconscious trying to tell you? How can you address this in your waking life?

- *Identifying potential gifts.* Our shadow attributes can often point us toward characteristics that can be of great benefit to us or the world. For example, envy may show you hidden goals you didn't know you wanted to pursue; anger may indicate a desire to fight injustice; impatience might indicate a passion for taking action that could be directed to a good cause; fear may highlight where you need more safety or boundaries; sadness may show you what you truly value.

  How would you rewrite one of your shadow traits so that it becomes a strength and reveals your gift to the world?

Remember, shadow work is a process. Be gentle with yourself as you explore these questions, and revisit them as your insights deepen over time.

WHEN OUR SHADOWS SLEEP, SO DO WE

Real-life outcomes of shadow work are profound. For example, someone struggling with insomnia due to perfectionism may discover, through shadow work, that this need for flawlessness stems from a childhood belief that mistakes equal failure. By reframing this belief and accepting their own humanity, they begin to release self-imposed pressure, ease their anxiety, and find sleep comes more naturally. Another person, plagued by recurring nightmares of being chased, might learn that the pursuer represents a fear of facing unresolved grief. Through journaling and therapy, they welcome their grieving self who had been lurking in the shadows, and over time the nightmares subside and sleep becomes restorative.

Shadow work isn't about "fixing" yourself—because the shadow within you is not a problem to be solved. Instead, it's about knowing yourself more fully. It's about welcoming the whole of who you are. When you take the time to explore and integrate the parts of yourself you've hidden away, you naturally enhance your emotional well-being and create the mental and emotional space needed for quality sleep.

In the end, shadow work reminds us that the parts of ourselves we fear the most are often the ones that hold the greatest potential for healing and growth. These are the parts that offer us the authenticity to live more fully and enjoyably. In a sense, our shadows are sometimes more "real" than the personas we present to the world. By facing our shadows, we not only transform our nights but also bring a new awareness to our waking lives—one that is lighter and freer of guilt. As this emotional burden lifts, both our days and our nights become richer, more peaceful, and more whole.

8

SOUND THERAPY AND SILENCE

DRIVING THROUGH THE SERENE AND SCORCHING DESERT NEAR Joshua Tree, California, you'd never guess that hidden among the sagebrush and spiny Joshua trees lies a structure that looks like it sprung to life from the pages of a sci-fi novel: the Integratron. Equal parts acoustic wonder and spiritual haven, its white dome, gleaming in the sunlight, appears like a futuristic mirage in the desolate desert, beckoning you, begging you to explore it.

I was there on the recommendation of a mentor in the fellowship program at the Andrew Weil Center for Integrative Medicine at The University of Arizona. He urged me to go there for a sound bath so I could experience the structure's anodyne capabilities. I was new to sound baths, but since I was deep into exploring alternative ways of healing and the Integratron was described as a "giant singing bowl for your soul," I was intrigued. So, on the hottest day in June, a few of my friends and I left for this otherworldly structure in the desert.

Constructed in 1954 by George Van Tassel, an aviation engineer who claimed the design was inspired by a combination of Nikola Tesla's electrical theories and instructions from extraterrestrials, the dome is oddly simple yet also transcendental. It was meant to be a time machine of sorts, but today, its primary claim to fame is its sound baths.

Inside, the Integratron felt serene and sacred. Warm wooden beams curved overhead like a soothing cocoon. There were no visible nails in the construction; the entire structure was assembled with perfect acoustics in mind. After climbing a tortuous and rather tenuous staircase, we reclined on mats arranged in a circle, with pillows and blankets to make the experience more comfortable. I noticed that everyone looked peaceful, almost like they were about to step into a collective dream that would transport them to an unknown, extraplanetary destination. I felt apprehensive and simultaneously intrigued.

The session began with a guide softly explaining the process. Crystal singing bowls, each tuned to a specific frequency, would be played in sequences meant to align with the body's energy centers, or chakras. Even though I was completely open to the experience, I was also skeptical. But I allowed myself to go with it. I closed my eyes as the first bowl began to hum.

At first, the sound was just that—a sound. But as it grew, the vibrations became something I could physically feel. I felt the reverberations gently nudging my body to relax. My chest, usually tight from the day's stress, felt like it was opening, letting in energy. Each bowl created a unique note, blending into a euphony that filled the entire dome. The sound didn't just wash over my body; it seemed to pass through me as if it were reading me, my anxiety, my story.

And then it happened: a strange, magical sensation of letting go and letting things be. I could feel my mind slow down, as though the frequencies were untangling things, untangling overthinking, untangling the issues that were troubling. My breathing deepened without effort.

My jaw unclenched. My body felt that it was levitating, as if I were being elevated by a behemoth force larger than I could fathom.

Later, I learned that the frequencies of the bowls are specifically tuned to promote relaxation and balance brain-wave activity, encouraging the kind of alpha and theta brain waves associated with deep meditation and restful sleep. But, for me, this was more than a balanced brain-wave activity; it was a spiritual and otherworldly experience. Yes, this experience could be explained scientifically, but it was also something more, something that I couldn't point to, something metaphysical and spiritual.

One woman in the group shared afterward that she'd struggled with chronic insomnia for years, but at that moment, she could feel her body surrendering to something close to rest, something that she could not necessarily explain, but something that allayed her anxiety and allowed her to sleep peacefully. She had not known rest like this before. She had become a poor sleeper after being hospitalized in the ICU for a protracted illness, but the acoustics in the Integratron made her feel like her sleep had normalized. She had slept in the Integratron, something she could never do elsewhere.

I didn't fall asleep during the sound bath, but when I arrived home, I felt relaxed and rejuvenated. That night, I had one of the best sleep experiences I'd had in months. The sound bath seemed to have unlocked something in me, clearing the noise of daily life and leaving behind a sense of stillness. When I feel anxiety or experience insomnia now, I remember that sound bath and the vibrations of the bowls, and my body begins to relax and let go.

The experience opened me up to the way sound can influence the body and mind. To the fact it can alter our outlook and perspective on life. To the way it can influence our sleep and sense of well-being. Luckily, you don't need to visit the Integratron to experience the benefits of sound therapy.

MUSIC AS MEDICINE

In his latest book, *I Heard There Was a Secret Chord,* the neuroscientist and musician Daniel J. Levitin explores how music interacts with our brain's networks, including the default mode network (DMN), to promote relaxation and facilitate sleep. The DMN is a network of interacting brain regions that becomes active during restful introspection and mind-wandering—when we're not focused on the external environment and specific tasks that we must accomplish. Essentially, absent attention to something, our brain "defaults" and our thoughts become unguided. It's a time for absentmindedness, for inward-directed thinking. Levitin's research has demonstrated that the switch to the DMN resides in the insula, a region in the brain where three of the four regions of the brain—frontal, parietal, and temporal—intersect. He has also showed that music can help us to enter this daydreaming state and engage in self-reflection, guiding the brain from active, task-oriented states to more restful ones.[1] This transition of the brain's activity is essential for winding down and preparing for sleep.

As Levitin suggests, music's rhythm and melody can synchronize with our biological processes, a phenomenon known as entrainment. For instance, slow-tempo music can align with and slow down our heart rate and breathing patterns, promoting a state of calm conducive to sleep. This synchronization helps shift the brain's activity from external task engagement to internal restfulness, engaging the DMN and paving the way for sleep. But the sweet spot, as Levitin suggests, is music that is both surprising and predictable. He argues that it should fall slightly to the "predictable side" to calm us, but not so much that it puts us to sleep or annoys us with its repetitiveness. The right balance of surprise and predictability helps restore focus and emotional balance during the day, resetting the mind after overstimulation. In turn, this state of calm alertness supports healthier sleep later, since we're entering the night less frazzled and more centered.

Ultimately, music serves as a distraction from stressors and intrusive thoughts that often hinder our ability to fall asleep. By focusing on soothing melodies, we divert attention from daily worries, allowing the DMN to facilitate a relaxed mental state. Slow-tempo, low-arousal music activates the parasympathetic system—the part responsible for rest, digestion, and recovery—lowering heart rate, blood pressure, and cortisol levels. Slow, rhythmic music, especially with a tempo around sixty beats per minute, can slow heart rate, lower blood pressure, and encourage deep, steady breathing. Over time, incorporating music into your nightly routine can lead to habit formation, where the brain associates certain music with relaxation and sleep, making it easier to transition into restfulness. Also, when we listen to music we like, it releases dopamine, a neurotransmitter associated with pleasure. This release not only enhances mood but also reduces anxiety, creating an optimal environment for the DMN to operate and promote sleep.

Beyond relaxation, music also shapes the brain through neuroplasticity, the brain's ability to rewire and adapt. Engaging with music, whether by listening, playing an instrument, or even humming, strengthens neural connections, especially in areas linked to emotion, memory, and learning. It can help "rewire" anxious patterns by reinforcing pathways associated with calmness and positive emotions. Over time, this repeated exposure to soothing or uplifting music can train the brain to respond to stress more resiliently. As Levitin reminds us, music isn't just a distraction from anxiety; it's a tool that actively reshapes the brain and nervous system, making relaxation and emotional balance more accessible in everyday life.[2]

SOUND THERAPY FOR INSOMNIA AND BETTER SLEEP

As Levitin and others have shown, sound has an undeniable impact on the human brain. This science is now being brought to bear in sleep medicine through sound therapy. Because our brains are deeply attuned to auditory stimuli, and because so many of the cues for sleep are modulated by the brain, sound therapy works. Like I experienced at the Integratron, specific sounds and frequencies can promote relaxation, reduce stress, and guide the brain into slower brain-wave states associated with deep sleep. It's like a sonic guide, gently leading your mind to a place of rest and allowing you to let go of your anxieties, fear, and restlessness.

One of the most buzzworthy innovations in sound therapy is binaural beats. These are audio tracks where two slightly different frequencies are played in each ear. For example, when your left ear hears a tone at 200 Hz and your right ear hears 210 Hz, your brain hears a third "beat" at the difference—in this case, 10 Hz.[3] That 10 Hz frequency aligns with brain waves linked to relaxation and light sleep. Binaural beats are thought to influence brain-wave activity, guiding your brain into specific states, such as delta waves, which are associated with slow-wave sleep. Listening through headphones is crucial because the beats rely on isolating each frequency to separate ears. Research is still evolving, but many studies suggest that binaural beats can improve relaxation and sleep onset.[4] In addition, it's noninvasive, drug-free, and easy to try, so there's nothing to lose.

If you've ever fallen asleep to your favorite playlist, you've already dabbled in and been introduced to the kind of music therapy Levitin was describing. This method involves using specific types of music to help you relax and prepare for sleep. Slow tempos are conducive to rest and sleep; music with sixty to eighty beats per minute mimics the natural rhythm of a relaxed heart rate and promotes sleep. Gentle, repetitive patterns without jarring changes are best. Opt for instrumental sounds as lyrics can be distracting. Piano, strings, or ambient sounds work particularly well. Music has been shown to reduce cortisol levels (the stress hormone) and activate the parasympathetic nervous system, which is responsible for calming our body.[5] Apps and streaming platforms now offer curated sleep playlists, making it easy to find the right soundscape for bedtime.

The future of sound therapy is exciting, as neuroscientists partner with innovative technology companies to redefine how we treat insomnia. There are some promising trends on the horizon. Imagine a bedtime app that uses AI to analyze your sleep patterns and tailors sound frequencies or music tracks to your unique needs. Personalized sound therapy is emerging, promising to make treatments even more effective and more relatable.

Devices such as headbands or earbuds designed for sleep therapy are becoming more advanced, as well. These gadgets can play binaural beats, white noise, or soothing music while tracking your sleep data for continuous improvement. Also, virtual reality sound therapy is just hitting the market. Imagine immersing yourself in a calming virtual forest, island, or beach, with 3D sound guiding you to relaxation. This multisensory approach could elevate sound therapy to new heights. Researchers are now also exploring how targeted sound therapies might be used to synchronize brain activity and address insomnia at its root. This could open doors to highly effective treatments with minimal side effects.

Sound therapy is easy to try and surprisingly effective for many people. A great number of my patients already use it and have found it to be both relaxing and effective for allaying anxiety linked to insomnia. There are many apps that offer binaural beats, guided sound meditations, and sleep-focused soundtracks. Create your "sound environment" by investing in a white noise machine or a high-quality speaker or headphones to play soothing sounds. White noise machines work by blending all audible frequencies together at equal intensity, creating a steady, neutral sound that masks sudden changes in the environment, like a door closing, traffic outside, or a partner shifting in bed. By smoothing over these peaks and valleys of noise, the brain no longer needs to stay half-alert for unexpected sounds, allowing the nervous system to relax into deeper, more continuous sleep. Even a fan or air purifier can serve as a source of calming background noise. Also, don't forget to set the mood, as this could create the perfect background. Candles and various scents, such as lavender, can elevate this experience to a film of sorts. Dim the lights, power down your screens, and let the sound guide you into rest. Like any new habit, sound therapy works best if it's used consistently. Use it nightly for a few weeks and notice how your body responds.

LISTENING TO THE SOUNDS OF YOUR OWN BRAIN

Perhaps the most interesting and idiosyncratic nontraditional method for treating insomnia resides within us, within our personal brain waves. Imagine lying in bed, wide awake, when instead of silence, you listen to music that's not just relaxing—it's uniquely you. That's the idea behind a fascinating innovation in music therapy: transforming the brain's electrical activity into soothing, custom-made soundscapes that are created when you are in a relaxed state. It's like composing a lullaby from the sounds your own brain makes and then using that recording to help you fall asleep at another time.

This technique involves recording your brain's EEG (electroencephalogram) waves, which reflect your brain's electrical activity, while you're relaxed and well-rested. These signals are then converted into music. Since EEG waves are associated with different states of mind—for example, slow delta waves are linked to deep sleep, while faster beta waves often appear when we're alert or stressed—by mapping these brain-wave patterns to specific musical tones or rhythms, the resulting music mirrors your brain in its relaxed state. As you listen, the music gradually encourages your brain to slow down, nudging it toward the calm, slower rhythms associated with sleep.

This form of music therapy is effective because our brain recognizes and responds to its own activity, creating a loop of self-regulation. Listening to music based on our brain waves can be inherently calming, helping reduce anxiety or racing thoughts that often accompany insomnia. Unlike generic playlists, this music reflects our unique neural activity, making it more effective at targeting what our brain needs in that moment. It is idiosyncratic to our own situation.

While this field is still emerging, early studies suggest that brain wave–based music therapy can help people fall asleep faster and experience deeper, more restorative sleep.[6] It's particularly promising for individuals with chronic insomnia or those who struggle with stress-induced sleeplessness. Some sleep clinics and specialized apps or devices offer this technology. You might need to visit a provider to have your EEG recorded, or you could explore home-based tools that use sensors to capture your brain activity and generate music in real time.[7]

SILENCE AS A SOLUTION

While music and binaural beats often get the spotlight for helping us drift off, silence—true, deep quiet—can also be powerful. Pico Iyer, in his book *Aflame: Learning from Silence*, shares how stepping into a world stripped of noise gave his restless mind something more precious than distraction: stillness. His visits to a silent Benedictine retreat in Big Sur, California, a trip he has made for decades, have allowed him to ponder challenges that he faced, such as a home burning down, a parent's death, and a daughter's diagnosis of cancer. In these retreats, he expected physical rest but also discovered a kind of inner reset. The monastery creates a nothingness in which its inhabitants become nothing; it offers an emptiness so that individuals can be filled up. In that hush, Iyer noticed the chatter in his head settling down, and a sense of clarity rising.[8] For some, especially those overstimulated by a noisy world, silence isn't just soothing; it's medicinal.

It invites the nervous system to finally exhale, making room for sleep to emerge naturally.

Music and silence, then, may seem like opposites. One fills the room, while the other clears it. One envelops, while the other takes away. But both can shape the space we fall asleep in. Music, especially slow and rhythmic, can soothe a racing mind, offering a gentle bridge from wakefulness to rest. Silence, on the other hand, allows us to meet ourselves without distraction, creating the stillness needed for the body to fully let go. Some nights call for melody, others for quiet. The key is learning which form of sound—or its absence—your nervous system needs to surrender to sleep that night.

9

HARNESSING THE POWER OF LIGHT AND DARK

Honestly, I never gave light and dark much thought, at least not until I became a sleep specialist and saw how deeply they shape the way we sleep. Growing up, I thought of them as switches: Light meant daytime hustle; darkness meant it was time to shut off. When I was a child, my parents would shut off the light switch in the bedroom that my twin sister and I shared. No dimmer, no slow acclimation to sleep. That was the start of the night, whether we were sleepy or not. But as I grew up, I realized that light and dark are not just passive backdrops to our lives. They're the directors, the quiet orchestrators behind the scenes shaping our energy, our moods, and the delicate surrender of sleep itself. We don't just live in light and dark; we live through them.

Many years ago, I traveled to a small, weathered coastal town in Rhode Island, one of those places where time seems to soften around the edges and stand still. There were no towering streetlamps, no neon signs blazing through the night. Just the low glow of porch lights and the moon's reflection stretching across the deep, black water. That night, something unusual happened. I fell asleep without a fight. No scrolling through endless headlines, no racing thoughts. It was as if my body, relieved to be freed from the tyranny of electric light, slipped naturally into a rhythm it had almost forgotten. It struck me then: We truly take light and dark for granted.

Science, of course, explains our relationship to light and dark beautifully. Exposure to natural darkness triggers the pineal gland to secrete melatonin, the hormone that signals to the body that it's time to rest. Artificial light, especially blue light, suppresses melatonin production, keeping the brain on alert when it should be winding down. It's not just a matter of feeling sleepy or not; it's about whether the fundamental gears of the body's circadian clock are turning smoothly or grinding against themselves.

But, as the theme of this book suggests, to reduce light and dark only to science misses something essential. Light and dark aren't only mechanical levers; they are metaphysical forces shaping not just our biology but our very experience of time, mood, mystery. Darkness invites introspection. It collapses the outer world so the inner one can expand. Sleep, then, is not merely a biological necessity but a nightly act of synchronicity with forces greater than us: a falling into the unknown, shielded by the soft cover of night.

I sometimes wonder if our collective sleep problems are not just about late-night scrolling or binge-watching but about a deeper estrangement from darkness itself. We've made darkness into something to be feared, warded off, pushed away with 60-watt bulbs. But maybe what we need is not more light at night but to reacquaint ourselves with darkness. We need to remember that the dark is not the enemy of life, but its partner. Without the night, there is no rest. Without rest, there is no renewal.

And so, now I try, imperfectly but intentionally, to let darkness back into my life. I dim the lights earlier. I allow the evening to settle instead of fighting it. Sometimes, I simply sit in the dark for a few minutes before bed, letting my mind adjust, letting my body *hear* the old cue: *It's time to cross over. Now. Allow it.* Sleep begins long before we lie down. It begins in our relationship with light, with dark. It is a quiet, ancient dialogue. A dialogue we are all still invited to join, if only we are willing to listen.

LET THERE BE LIGHT

When was the last time you truly experienced darkness—real, complete darkness? For most of human history, our sleep was intimately tied to the rise and fall of the sun, what we call standard time. The glow of candles or moonlight was the dimmest illumination we encountered after sunset. Then, in 1879, Thomas Edison changed everything. The incandescent light bulb did more than illuminate homes, factories, and street: It transformed the very structure of time. Before electricity, people lived by a segmented sleep pattern, often waking in the middle of the night for quiet reflection, prayer, sex, and other social interactions before drifting into a second phase of sleep. This biphasic sleep, a common feature of preindustrial societies, began to erode as artificial light extended the day into night. It was as if the day became one long stretch, with the brain unable to distinguish its natural circadian cues. No longer bound to the setting sun—hooray!—people could work, read, and socialize far past natural bedtime. As we now know, this came with a cost with which we are still grappling and reeling.

The historian A. Roger Ekirch, in his book *At Day's Close: Night in Times Past,* argues that artificial light disrupted this natural rhythm of "segmented sleep."[1] As candles became cheaper, and, later, gas and electric lights spread, night was no longer the boundary it used to be. Activities extended into the evening, and the cultural norm shifted toward a single, consolidated sleep period. Before this, darkness had dictated sleep; it told the body when to shut down. But once the night became illuminated, we started to squeeze sleep into one continuous block—shorter, more compressed, and often more restless. Sleep stopped being a slow unfolding of dusk into dawn and became something to get over with so we could get on with our lives. Ironically, forcing sleep into one consolidated stretch may have made sleep feel more fragile. We were trying to override thousands of years of coevolution with the planet. Instead of embracing our body's rhythm, we started fighting it and calling it a disorder when it pushed back. Ekirch poignantly notes, "By turning night into day, modern technology has helped to obstruct our oldest path to the human psyche," highlighting how the loss of darkness has distanced us from introspective moments once integral to our nightly routine. In many ways, the modern sleep crisis began with the flick of a switch.

It's entirely possible that modern insomnia is a remnant of something older—an echo of our lost biphasic sleep. Before industrialization, waking up in the middle of the night wasn't pathological; it was expected. What we now label as "middle-of-the-night insomnia" may be a biological holdover from that earlier rhythm. Instead of being broken, maybe our sleep is trying to follow a pattern it once knew well but in a culture that no longer makes space for it. Perhaps the sleepless hours at 3:00 a.m. aren't a flaw but a forgotten invitation to rest differently.

The German historian Wolfgang Schivelbusch, in his book *Disenchanted Night*, describes how the industrialization of light changed not only how people lived but also how they perceived darkness itself. Once a familiar and natural part of existence, night was increasingly seen as an obstacle to work, to entertainment—something to be conquered and vanquished. As gaslight gave way to electricity, darkness retreated further, and the nocturnal world of dreams and silence was increasingly displaced by the hum and buzz of modern life. "Night," Schivelbusch writes, "was no longer a pause but a mere continuation of the day."[2]

This shift came at a brutal cost, which we are still paying. Sleep, once governed by natural circadian rhythms, became subject to the demands of productivity. The blue-rich spectrum of electric light, particularly in the fluorescent and LED bulbs that followed Edison's invention, interfered with the body's production of melatonin, the "vampire" hormone that signals the onset of sleep. As nighttime became brighter, insomnia and sleep disturbances became more common. The body, still biologically attuned to the natural cycles of sunrise and sunset, struggled to adjust to a world where darkness was banished by us.

DANCING TO THE CIRCADIAN RHYTHM

At the heart of our body's internal clock is the circadian rhythm, a roughly twenty-four-hour cycle that governs not only our sleep-wake patterns but also our metabolism, mood, and even immune function. This rhythm is regulated by a small group of neurons in the hypothalamus called the suprachiasmatic nucleus (SCN). And what causes the SCN to keep time? Light.

When light enters our eyes, special cells in the retina (called intrinsically photosensitive retinal ganglion cells, or ipRGCs) send signals to the SCN. Bright, blue-rich light—like that from the sun or electronic screens—tells the brain that it's morning, that it's time to start the day. This suppresses the release of melatonin, the vampire hormone that helps us feel sleepy, from the pineal gland. In contrast, darkness signals the brain to ramp up melatonin production, preparing us for rest. Modern life, however, has disrupted this delicate balance. Exposure to artificial light at night confuses the brain into thinking it's still daytime, delaying melatonin release and shifting the body's natural sleep-wake cycle. The result? Insomnia and a delayed sleep phase. Difficulty falling asleep, fragmented sleep, and groggy mornings.

Our ancestors instinctively aligned their lives with the natural patterns of light and darkness. Agricultural societies rose with the sunrise and rested shortly after sunset, their bodies attuned to the rhythms of nature. Many ancient cultures even had rituals that emphasized the importance of light and darkness. Ancient Egyptians revered the sun god Ra, understanding the sun's life-giving power. Early morning sunlight was considered cleansing and energizing. In some Tibetan Buddhist practices, monks would spend days in total darkness to promote inner stillness and mental clarity. These practices weren't just spiritual; they were deeply restorative. Exposure to bright natural light during the day helped regulate their circadian rhythms, while the absence of artificial light at night ensured high-quality sleep.

In our modern day-to-day life, there are practical ways to harness light and darkness for better sleep and rest. Embrace morning light, especially if your schedule is off kilter from travel, shift work, or other life demands. Natural light in the morning is the most powerful way to set your internal clock. Studies have shown that exposure to sunlight within the first hour of waking can help you feel more alert during the day. It can also strengthen your circadian rhythm, making it easier to fall asleep at night and improve mood by increasing serotonin production.

To reset your clock, spend fifteen to thirty minutes outdoors shortly after waking, even if it's cloudy. Open your curtains wide to let natural light flood your space. Consider a light therapy box (10,000 lux) if natural sunlight is limited in your area or during seasons when the sky is often overcast. Light in the morning is useful. Use it. Harness it. Smartly.

Just as we should embrace light in the morning, we should dim the lights in the evening to signal to our bodies that it's time to wind down. Bright, artificial lights at night suppress melatonin, tricking the brain into staying alert. Instead, use warm, low-intensity lights in the evening. Switch to lamps with dimmable settings or amber light bulbs. Avoid screens (or use blue-light filters) one to two hours before bed. Blue light is the most disruptive to melatonin production, although the amount of light and its intensity, or lux, is probably more important than wavelength (color).

Lux is a way of measuring how much light reaches our eyes. It's not just about how bright a light looks, but how much it can influence our body. For example, bright daylight can hit 10,000 lux (even on a cloudy day you can get 1,000 lux), while indoor office lighting usually hovers around 300 to 500 lux. In the evening, try to keep the lights in your home at 100 lux or less. In addition to the intensity (lux), the exposure and duration matter as well. Even moderate light, if you're exposed to it long enough or at the wrong time (like late at night), can delay melatonin and disrupt your sleep. So, whether it's morning sunlight or dim screens at bedtime, your body is constantly listening to the light around you and responding.

Darkness is essential for deep, restorative sleep. Even a sliver of light during the night, such as the glow of a clock, the light under a door, or the blue glow of a charger, can disrupt sleep cycles by interfering with melatonin production. As mentioned above, your eyes are wired with special light-sensitive cells called intrinsically photosensitive retinal ganglion cells that send signals straight to your brain's sleep-wake clock—the suprachiasmatic nucleus. Even low levels of light (less than 10 lux) can delay melatonin production and shift our sleep cycle. One study showed that exposure to room light before bed suppressed melatonin secretion by approximately ninety minutes compared to dim light. Light intensity while sleeping should not exceed 1 lux, which is essentially pitch-black.[3] In short, blue light (wavelength) matters less than light intensity and duration, although we should still turn off our tablets and other "active" screens at least one to two hours before sleep.

Light at night can also make your sleep shallower and fragment your REM cycles. Studies have found that even one night of sleeping with moderate light exposure (100 lux) increased heart rate and insulin resistance the next morning.[4] So, yes, that seemingly innocent glow from your neighbor's porch light or your partner's late-night phone or e-reader session could be sabotaging your rest and metabolism.

In contrast, reading a paper book under dim, warm light has very little impact on melatonin. Some sleep experts take a stricter stance—recommending that the bed be reserved only for sleep and sex to strengthen the brain's association between bed and rest. Yet many people find that brief, calm reading under dim light can gently ease the transition to sleep. The key is not the activity itself, but its quality: quiet, screen-free, and done with mindful awareness of drowsiness. In fact, it can be part of a relaxing bedtime ritual that supports our body's natural sleep rhythm. A landmark study from Harvard found that using a tablet for four hours before bed suppressed melatonin production by about 55 percent and delayed its rise by more than an hour and a half compared to reading a print book under dim light. Not only that, but participants also felt less sleepy at bedtime and had reduced REM sleep. And the following morning, they were groggier and had lower alertness compared to those who read physical books.[5]

To protect your sleep from unwanted light, the first step is making your bedroom as dark as possible. Blackout curtains can be a total game-changer; they block out streetlights, headlights, and even early morning sun if you're a late sleeper. If curtains aren't an option, a well-fitting sleep mask is a solid alternative. Just ensure that it seals well around the nose to prevent light leaks. It also helps to unplug or cover up any glowing electronics; those tiny LED lights on chargers or alarm clocks might seem harmless, but they can still stimulate your brain's alertness. You can purchase inexpensive light-dimming stickers to cover them.

ADVANCED AND DELAYED SLEEP PHASE SYNDROMES

In my practice, I treat a variety of circadian rhythm disturbances. When someone is coming to see me because they're having trouble sleeping, I can often make an educated guess about their problem based on their age and the time of day they scheduled their appointment.

Patients with advanced sleep phase syndrome (ASPS) are morning larks and are usually elderly. They feel sleepy early in the evening—often long before their peers—and awaken exceptionally early in the morning. Their internal clocks appear to be set several hours ahead of the norm, and they often complain of missing out on evening social events because they just can't stay awake. They come for the first appointments of the day because they've already been up for hours.

In contrast, patients with delayed sleep phase syndrome (DSPS) make appointments for late in the day and are often younger. These individuals are night owls and can struggle with falling asleep, often not doing so until very late at night or early morning, which can result in a late wake-up time that is out of sync with societal expectations. They are often late for morning appointments, classes, or work.

If you are a morning lark (those with ASPS), your goal is to delay your internal clock so that you can stay up longer to enjoy those social activities you may have missed out on. Evening light exposure can help. By safely exposing yourself to gentle, controlled light in the early evening—about 2,000 to 10,000 lux for thirty to sixty minutes, or by spending time outdoors two to three hours before your intended bedtime—you can help shift your internal clock later and ease the symptoms of advanced sleep phase syndrome. This can slow the onset of sleepiness by delaying the drop in your core body temperature that signals your body is preparing for sleep. And this, in turn, nudges your melatonin onset to a later time, aligning your sleep schedule more closely with your desired routine.

In addition to getting early evening light, it will also help you to get some early morning light, but the timing is important and will involve doing a little math. First, you'll need to determine when your minimum core body temperature (CBTmin) happens. This naturally happens roughly two hours prior to your current "natural" wake-up time, which is the time you would wake up without an alarm. For example, if you naturally wake at 4:00 a.m., your CBTmin happens around 2:00 a.m. To help nudge that time to be later, you'll want to get about twenty to thirty minutes of exposure to bright light (10,000 lux) just before your CBTmin time, which means around 1:30 a.m. Since this timing is often in the middle of the dark night for most of the world, you'll need to do this with a light box rather than natural sunlight. You can return to bed afterward if you're able, and the process usually needs to be repeated daily for a week or two before your body clock gradually shifts to a later schedule.

If you are a night owl (those with DSPS), your goal is to advance your internal clock. Bright light exposure in the morning is crucial—think of it as resetting the alarm clock in your brain. By immersing yourself in natural sunlight or using a light therapy box (10,000 lux) soon after waking, you signal to your body that it's time to be alert. Start with twenty to thirty minutes when you wake up. Since you don't want to do this too early (as it can delay your sleep even further), you'll need to do a bit of math too, just like those with ASPS, but your instructions will be different.

First, you'll need to determine when your minimum core body temperature (CBTmin) happens. As I said before, this naturally happens roughly two hours prior to your current "natural" wake-up time. Let's say if you don't have to set the alarm clock, you wake up on your own at 11:00 a.m. That means your CBTmin happens around 9:00 a.m. To advance your circadian rhythm, meaning to try and naturally bump yourself in the direction of going to sleep earlier and waking earlier, you'll want to get direct sunlight just after your CBTmin. In this case, that means just after 9:00 a.m. If you do it before then, you may actually delay evening sleep further.

Night owls can further help to shift their circadian rhythms by limiting exposure to bright light in the evening. If the sun is still bright in the evening, like it is in summers where I live in California, wear sunglasses at night. I'm a night owl, and I routinely wear sunglasses in the evening during the summer months, and it helps my circadian rhythm stay on track.

In both cases, for morning larks and night owls, you can work with this light exposure until you find a time that best suits you. My patients are both astounded and excited when I help them calculate their core body temperature and timed exposure to light. They think it's some type of magic. Yes, it's science, but it's also magical when it works.

Sleep is not just about what happens in the dark; it's also about what happens in the light. By intentionally embracing light during the day and welcoming darkness at night, we align ourselves with the natural rhythms of the universe and our own bodies. In the alchemy of sleep, light and darkness are the catalysts. When balanced, they create the conditions for deep, restorative rest. By reclaiming these ancient forces and integrating them with modern science, we can transform our nights.

EMBRACING THE SACRED POWER OF DARKNESS

Beyond the physical benefits for sleep, darkness has a psychological and spiritual dimension. Quiet, dark spaces allow the mind to slow down, promoting relaxation and introspection. Ancient cultures understood this well: Darkness was a time for dreams, inner work, renewal. Incorporating intentional periods of darkness into your day—whether through meditation in a dimly lit room or a calming bedtime routine—can help you transition into a restful state. Sleep is not a switch that can be turned on and off. I hope that by now you realize that sleep is a relationship. Speak with it. Spend time with it. Let it guide you intuitively.

Think of light and dark as two ancient, eternal partners. Light, vibrant and energizing, carries with it the promise of a new beginning. It awakens our senses, fills us with vitality, and helps us align with the world around us. In contrast, darkness is not merely the absence of light: It is a time for introspection, for surrendering to rest. Our modern lives, with their constant glow from screens and artificial lighting, often blur these natural transitions. It's as if we've forgotten the wisdom of nature's own rhythms.

As the sun retreats and twilight descends, we are gifted with a sacred invitation to slow down. This is the time to honor the coming darkness as a cherished ally. Dimming the lights can be a meditation in itself: a conscious, deliberate act of letting go. In these moments, the flicker of a candle can evoke ancient imagery of quiet contemplation, of inner peace. It's a time to reflect on the day's experiences, to release what no longer serves you, to prepare for a night of restorative sleep. Here, the darkness is not frightening; it's nurturing. It invites you to connect with silence, with yourself.

At its core, sleep is a return to our most authentic state. When we allow ourselves to surrender fully to the night, free from the distractions of artificial light, we embrace a process that is both physiological and profoundly existential. It's as though by honoring the natural cycle of light and dark, we are also acknowledging the cycles of growth, decay, and rebirth within ourselves.

In many spiritual traditions, darkness is revered as a time for introspection and healing. It's during these quiet hours, these still hours, that our inner light can shine the brightest, illuminating parts of ourselves that are often hidden in the glare of day-to-day life. Embracing the dark can be an act of self-compassion, a deliberate choice to nurture your inner being.

Sleep, then, doesn't begin when we close our eyes. It begins when we let the night back in. So, let it in, because the dark is just the night. We don't need to be afraid of it.

10

ADJUSTING YOUR DIET TO SUPPORT SLEEP

DURING MY INTERNSHIP YEAR IN INTERNAL MEDICINE, months before my car accident and before I began my residency in neurology, my diet was a disaster: microwave dinners from Trader Joe's late at night (not horrible, but not optimal, either), protein bars that tasted like compressed cardboard (before they actually tasted good), and enough coffee during night calls to kill a small animal. I'd scarf something down during charting or rounds, usually while standing, barely tasting it. And somehow, I was always starving at 2:00 a.m., jittery from caffeine but crashing from sugar. My sleep became shallow and unpredictable. I'd lie down exhausted but felt wired, my stomach churning, my mind racing. Since then, I've learned better, especially when it comes to food that improves my sleep.

The connection between diet and sleep is old. In ancient traditions, diets were carefully aligned with natural rhythms, emphasizing balance, seasonality, and foods that nurtured both body and mind. These ancient dietary practices often prioritized sleep-friendly ingredients and rituals. In contrast, modern dietary habits, which are shaped by fast-paced lifestyles, processed foods, and irregular eating patterns, have introduced significant disruptions to sleep quality. This chapter explores how ancient wisdom guided dietary choices to promote restful sleep and how modern diets often undermine this vital process.

ANCIENT HEALING SYSTEMS AND SLEEP

Ancient healing systems, such as Ayurveda and Traditional Chinese Medicine (TCM), understood the profound influence of food on sleep. They viewed diet as both preventive and curative, capable of harmonizing the body's energy systems to foster deep, restorative rest.

Ayurveda classifies food by how it influences the *doshas*—*vata*, *pitta*, and *kapha*—and by its energetic qualities known as *gunas*. One's dominant dosha, evident in recurring patterns of digestion, sleep, mood, and stress response, guides which gunas (whether *sattvic*, *rajasic*, or *tamasic*) support balance and which disturb it. For promoting sleep, Ayurveda emphasizes sattvic foods that are light, fresh, and calming. Think warm milk, almonds, ghee, and rice: substances that are ideal for preparing the body for rest. Consuming easily digestible meals before sunset is considered essential to avoiding digestive strain that could disrupt sleep. Warm, spiced drinks with ingredients such as nutmeg or cardamom are used to calm the mind and balance vata, which often drives insomnia. Ayurveda also prescribes specific foods for each dosha. For instance, grounding and warm foods such as root vegetables and soups are recommended for vata insomnia, while cooling foods such as cucumber and mint are ideal for pitta-related sleep disturbances.

In Traditional Chinese Medicine, the relationship between food and sleep revolves around maintaining the smooth flow of qi and supporting organ systems. TCM emphasizes the health of the digestive system, or "middle burner," for optimal sleep. Foods that are warm, cooked, and easy to digest such as congee or soups support these organs and prevent nighttime disruptions. Foods and teas infused with sleep-promoting herbs such as jujube seeds (*suan zao ren*) and lotus seeds are used to calm the *shen* (spirit). Traditional diets align with the seasons, incorporating cooling foods in summer and warming foods in winter to balance yin and yang. Eating seasonally is believed to harmonize the body's internal clock, supporting better sleep.

Ancient Greeks and Romans also valued light evening meals with foods such as lentils, honey, and figs, which are rich in sleep-promoting nutrients such as magnesium and tryptophan. They avoided heavy, oily foods late in the day to prevent digestive discomfort. Their diets were largely Mediterranean in nature—abundant in fruits, vegetables, whole grains, olive oil, and fish—foods that naturally supported stable energy and better sleep. Wine was often enjoyed in moderation and sometimes diluted with water, not as indulgence but ritual, helping the body and mind transition from the labors of the day to the quiet of the night. Even then, eating was understood not just as nourishment but as a rhythm aligned with light, rest, and the turning of the day.

THE MESS OF THE MODERN MEAL

In contrast, modern dietary practices, while convenient, often work against the body's natural rhythms, disrupting sleep in profound ways. Processed foods, irregular mealtimes, and stimulants have become commonplace, contributing to widespread sleep issues. Modern Western diets are loaded with refined sugars and carbohydrates. These cause spikes and crashes in blood sugar levels that can lead to fragmented sleep or waking in the middle of the night. In addition, artificial additives, including MSG and certain food dyes such as Red 40, Yellow 5, and Yellow 6, can overstimulate the nervous system, making it more difficult to wind down for sleep.[1]

The German historian Wolfgang Schivelbusch argues that stimulants such as coffee and sugar didn't just change diets—they changed the rhythms of life.[2] Before the explosion of stimulants in Europe (especially during the Industrial Revolution), life followed a much slower, more natural pace, synced to daylight and bodily needs. Sleep was deeper, longer, more attuned to darkness. But once coffee, tea, and sugar became widespread, they fueled longer workdays, sharper mental focus, and a push toward being "awake" longer than nature intended. Sleep became something to "manage," an obstacle to productivity rather than a vital part of life. The rise of stimulants that Schivelbusch describes fractured the old relationship people had with sleep. Sleep shifted from being a natural, sacred rhythm to something you tried to cut down, squeeze in, control. In a way, modern insomnia isn't just a personal failing or a medical problem. It's a cultural invention. We built a world and mind that runs on speed and stimulation, then wondered why we can't shut them off at night.

In addition, in this modern "tired but wired" age, or what has been referred to as the "twired" age, when we don't obtain enough sleep, the balance between two key appetite hormones—leptin and ghrelin—goes completely haywire. Leptin, which signals to our brain that we're full, drops. Meanwhile, ghrelin, the hormone that screams, "I'm starving!" rises. Adding to this maelstrom are endocannabinoids, chemicals produced by the body that are akin to cannabis. Sleep loss increases the levels of these chemicals, in addition to the already mentioned ghrelin, which doubly stimulate our appetite. The result? We're not only hungrier but less likely to feel satisfied after eating. It's a perfect hormonal storm for overeating.

I remember during residency, after too many twenty-eight-hour call shifts, I'd find myself in front of the hospital vending machine at 3:00 a.m., staring down a Snickers bar like it was life-saving medicine. I wasn't even truly hungry—it was pure, sleep-deprived biology. And studies back this up: People who consistently sleep less than six hours a night tend to eat more calories, especially from carbohydrates and fats, and have a more difficult time losing weight.[3] It's a vicious cycle, too: Weight gain can lead to poor sleep, which leads to more weight gain. Sleep isn't just rest; it's metabolism's secret weapon.

The widespread use of caffeine in coffee (as I know too well from my residency years), energy drinks, and sodas also significantly affects sleep quality. While ancient diets often included calming herbal teas, modern diets are more likely to rely on stimulants to combat fatigue, creating a vicious cycle of poor sleep and energy dependence.

Unlike ancient practices of aligning meals with the sun, modern lifestyles involve late-night eating or skipping meals altogether. Eating heavy or greasy foods late in the evening can strain digestion and disrupt sleep. The body is forced to work on digestion when it should be focusing on repair and rejuvenation. Moreover, the heat that is generated with this metabolism makes it more difficult to sleep as the body requires a cool environment to induce sleep. Also, constant grazing throughout the day can dysregulate insulin levels and disturb the body's internal clock, making it harder to establish a regular sleep schedule. While alcohol is often used as a sleep aid, its effects are deceptive. It may help people fall asleep faster (due to its short half-life), but it disrupts REM sleep, leading to poorer overall rest.

Several studies have shown that the type of food we select to eat is often determined by the amount of sleep that we obtained. In the sleep-deprived setting, studies have shown that the brain's reward centers (using an fMRI to track increased activity in certain portions of the brain) are more active in response to high sugar and fat foods. When sleep-deprived, the participants chose food that was high caloric and not healthy as opposed to when they obtained restful sleep.[4] In this scenario, not only are the reward centers affected but so is the prefrontal cortex, which is involved in executive function (planning, prioritizing, making decisions, and controlling impulses). In contrast, our more primal brain, namely the amygdala and other deep limbic structures, goes into overdrive. It gets more reactive, more emotional, and less rational, like our inner caveman taking the wheel while our prefrontal cortex naps in the car. As a result, with sleep deprivation, not only are we selecting foods that are desirable but not healthy for us, but we are also not reasoning why we made such a poor choice. We've reverted to being children who want something now, with no care for the dire consequences later. Although this relationship is complex and other factors are involved, data from the past fifty years implies that the rise in obesity coincides with the reduction in sleep time, which is understandable, given what we now know.[5]

THE BAD NEWS ABOUT ALCOHOL

Alcohol is woven into nearly every culture: a social lubricant, a marker of celebration, and often a quiet companion to the end of the day. Our rituals, from dinners to weddings to after-work gatherings, are frequently arranged around it, although this is changing as more people abstain from it due to its harmful effects. Yet the same substance that helps us unwind can easily disrupt the very rest we seek. The timing and amount matter: A single drink with dinner may have little effect, but alcohol consumed within a few hours of bedtime shortens REM sleep and fragments the night. Even the type plays a role: Darker spirits and red wine, which are rich in congeners (chemicals responsible for the taste and smell of alcohol that are harder to metabolize and are associated with hangovers), tend to produce more restlessness than lighter options such as clear spirits or diluted wine. Over time, what feels like relaxation can subtly erode the body's capacity for deep, restorative sleep.

Alcohol, which is widely consumed as a "nightcap," reduces REM sleep and causes awakenings throughout the night. It can also cause nocturia due to its diuretic properties, meaning you'll awaken to urinate, perhaps once or, more likely, many times. Alcohol might feel like a sleep aid—and at first glance, it kind of is. That glass (or two) of wine might help you fall asleep faster because it depresses the central nervous system, making you drowsy. But here's the catch: While alcohol can knock you out quickly, the sleep it provides is shallow, fragmented, and chemically altered. It's like slipping into a counterfeit version of rest. It's a kind of rest that leaves your brain foggy, your memory dulled, your body unrefreshed.

Research has consistently shown that alcohol suppresses REM sleep, which is critical for memory consolidation, emotional regulation, and learning. Numerous studies have revealed that even moderate doses of alcohol reduce REM early in the night and cause REM to rebound, meaning more REM later in the night, often in a more chaotic, dream-intense form. This rebound is also when people tend to wake up—tossing, turning, or sweating—as the sedative effect wears off and the body tries to rebalance.[6]

I often offer this example to my younger clients to explain how alcohol is not helping them. Let's say you're a college student who had a few drinks to relax the night before an exam. You fell asleep quickly, sure, but your brain spent the night skipping over the deeper stages of learning-related sleep. Without quality REM sleep, the facts you studied aren't efficiently transferred from short-term storage (hippocampus) to long-term memory (neocortex). The next day, you feel groggy, your reaction time is off, and your ability to retrieve information is frustratingly fuzzy. In sleep research terms, your brain missed its chance to "replay" and reinforce the material, and you're left without access to the information you need for your exam.

In short, alcohol disrupts the architecture of sleep. It slashes REM sleep and causes more frequent awakenings in the second half of the night. And the more you drink, the more exaggerated these effects become. So, while it may feel like a nightcap that helps you drift off, it steals the kind of restorative sleep you need most, especially when you're trying to perform, think clearly, or recall something important.

WHAT TO EAT AND WHEN TO EAT IT

There's no single food or supplement that guarantees a perfect night's sleep. Diet is just one thread in a much larger tapestry that includes light, stress, movement, and emotional balance. A good goal is to stabilize your energy and promote calm, not to induce sleep outright through food. Individual differences matter, too. For example, those who are sensitive to sugar may find that even a seemingly healthy bedtime snack, such as a banana, can trigger a blood sugar spike and subsequent crash that disrupts rest. Still, what and when we eat can gently nudge the body toward rest, especially when aligned with its natural rhythms. Drawing from both ancient wisdom and modern nutritional science, the following foods are known to support sleep:

- Warm milk contains tryptophan, which supports serotonin and melatonin production.
- Almonds are rich in magnesium, a mineral that relaxes muscles and calms the nervous system.
- Honey stabilizes blood sugar levels and aids in tryptophan release.
- Herbal teas, such as chamomile and valerian, calm the nervous system and promote relaxation.
- Bananas contain magnesium, potassium, and B6 to aid in muscle relaxation.
- Complex carbohydrates, such as sweet potato, can stabilize blood sugar levels and our sleep due to their high fiber content.

Conversely, the following foods can interfere with sleep:

- Caffeine stimulates the central nervous system due to its relatively long half-life, delaying sleep onset.
- Spicy foods, common in late-night snacking, can cause indigestion and raise body temperature.

- High-fat meals, which are associated with fast food and heavy dinners, delay digestion and may trigger acid reflux.
- Simple carbohydrates, such as white bread and bagels, can cause more sleep-maintenance insomnia, meaning you'll wake up more throughout the night.

To improve sleep, then, we can draw on ancient dietary wisdom and common sense while adapting it to modern lifestyles. Timing matters. Align meals with natural light cycles, eating the largest meal midday and a lighter, easily digestible dinner. Simplify ingredients. Prioritize whole, unprocessed foods over complex, additive-laden meals. Have an evening ritual in mind. Incorporate calming drinks such as herbal teas or warm milk as part of a wind-down routine. And, lastly, minimize stimulants, reducing caffeine and sugar, especially in the afternoon and evening hours. By merging the balance and intentionality of ancient diets with the accessibility of modern nutrition, you can reestablish the link between food and sleep, reclaiming rest.

My diet has changed drastically since I began my fellowship in sleep medicine (and, later, my fellowship in integrative medicine), and I'm deeply grateful for that shift. I hope you experience a similar transformation.

11

SLEEP AS A LITTLE DEATH

I REMEMBER LYING IN BED ONE NIGHT, NOT QUITE ASLEEP BUT not fully awake either, when it struck me: Sleep feels a little like dying, but in a strangely comforting way. My body was heavy, the room faded at the edges, Mazzy Star's dreamy and hazy track "Mary of Silence" was quietly playing on the stereo. I had this fleeting sense that I was dissolving. It wasn't dramatic. It wasn't morbid, either. It was like slipping out of form, out of identity, out of this world. It was peaceful, almost weightless, and for a moment I thought, "Maybe this is what it's like to die—just a quiet unhooking from the world, a temporary pause." It wasn't frightening; it wasn't suicidal ideation; it made me feel more present, more aware of how delicate and mysterious this nightly ritual really is.

In the introduction, I described how I was driving alone through the desert and drifted into sleep, waking inside the wreckage of my car. For a few seconds, maybe longer, I hovered between worlds—the one I knew and the one that almost took me. That moment altered everything I thought I understood about sleep, awareness, and what it means to "come back." Sleep and death are more similar than we'd like to think. It may sound grim to think like this, but it can also be calming to approach sleep and death in this way and on their own terms.

THE RAINBOW BODY IN TIBETAN BUDDHISM

Every night, we surrender to unconsciousness, a groundlessness, drifting beyond the boundaries of time, space, self. In deep sleep, we cease to exist as we know ourselves: no memories, no identity, just a formless awareness hovering in the void. And then, just as effortlessly, just as suddenly, just like that, through no action of our own, we return. This nightly disappearance is more than just a biological process. It's a rehearsal for the great dissolution that awaits us all: death. As the Buddhist teacher Pema Chödrön astutely suggests, "When groundlessness has become familiar territory for us, the ultimate groundlessness of death will no longer feel so threatening."[1] This every-night groundlessness is akin to death. In fact, Chödrön continues, "the experiences of dying, going through the intermediate state [the bardo], and taking a new birth [in the Buddhist sense] are said to match closely the daily process of falling asleep, dreaming, and waking up the next day."[2]

Treating sleep as a "little death" is comforting. It's a way of letting go—of our problems, of our baggage, of our ego—and becoming dead to the world, at least for the night. Similarly, thinking of death as sleep makes it more comforting and more familiar. We succumb. We lay down our arms. We make the unfamiliar more familiar. We take the horror out of the unknown.

In Tibetan Buddhism, sleep is more than rest; it is training for death. The rainbow body phenomenon, in which a realized master dissolves into pure light after dying, represents the culmination of this training. The rainbow body has been described as "the shrinkage and disappearance of a human body within a short time after death accompanied by paranormal phenomena such as unusual emanations of light and altered atmospheric conditions in the locality of the deceased."[3] But what does it mean to transform one's body into light? And could our nightly descent into sleep offer clues about how consciousness moves through death?

Tibetan teachings describe the process of dying as a gradual dissolution of the elements—earth, water, fire, wind, and space—until what remains is pure awareness. This mirrors what happens in deep sleep. The senses withdraw, and the body feels heavy, just as it does in the early stages of death. The mind detaches, thoughts slow then vanish, resembling the disorientation of dying. Consciousness fades into emptiness. In deep sleep, we enter a space beyond thought, much like the "clear light" state described in the *Bardo Thödol* (*The Tibetan Book of the Dead*).

In both sleep and death, the ego dissolves. If one can maintain awareness during sleep, Tibetan masters suggest, one can do the same in death, navigating it consciously rather than being swept away. This is the foundation of dream yoga, a practice in which sleep becomes a tool for awakening (see more about that in chapter 5). But what about the corporeal body? This is where the rainbow body comes in.

In 1872, a Tibetan master named Nyala Pema Dündul reportedly performed a feat that defies conventional understanding. At the time of his death, his body did not decay. Instead, it began to shrink, slowly dissolving over several days, until all that remained were his hair and fingernails. These were the only parts of the body said to lack energy channels, or *tsa*. His followers witnessed a strange luminosity filling the space where his body had been. This was not an isolated event; many high-level Dzogchen practitioners have been recorded as undergoing commensurate transformations.

Similarly, in 1998, Khenpo A Chö, a highly respected Tibetan Buddhist master, renowned for his deep meditative realization and devotion to the Dzogchen teachings, passed under similar circumstances.

Monastic witnesses and disciples reported that his body exhibited signs of the rainbow body phenomenon: His body gradually shrunk over the course of days, emanating light, and eventually leaving behind little more than hair and nails.

Tibetan Buddhism teaches that the physical body is a condensation of light, a denser form of energy that can be reabsorbed into its original essence. Through meditation, awareness in sleep, and mastery over the mind, the illusion of solidity dissolves, revealing the body's true nature. The rainbow body, then, is not a magic trick but the natural unfolding of an awakened being's realization. From a sleep medicine perspective, the rainbow body raises profound questions about the continuum of consciousness across sleep, dreaming, and death. While this "body" remains outside the scope of empirical science, these experiences encourage exploration between contemplative traditions and modern neuroscience, inviting further inquiry into the nature of awareness, sleep, and human potential.

SURRENDERING CONSCIOUSNESS

Sleep, in this framework, is not just a passive state but an opportunity. Every night, we undergo a miniature version of this dissolution: Our identity disappears, the body becomes inert, and consciousness merges into something beyond form. If we could remain aware in this process, Tibetan teachings suggest, we might begin to glimpse the light behind the illusion of solidity. This is the reason advanced practitioners use sleep as a gateway. Through lucid dreaming, dream yoga, and meditation, they prepare themselves for the final sleep that is death. If we learn to dissolve our mental grasp on form while alive, we may find that, at death, there is nothing to hold on to: only light, only vastness, only the boundless awareness that was always there.

The idea of dissolving into light may sound unattainable, reserved for Himalayan mystics. But the practice of awareness in sleep is available to me, to you, to everyone. Every night, as we slip into unconsciousness, we touch the same mystery that awaits us in death. By engaging with this process consciously, we may begin to loosen our grip on form, on identity, on the illusion of separateness. Perhaps the rainbow body is not just about leaving this world in a burst of light. Perhaps it's about realizing, even while alive, that we were never as solid as we seemed. We never were.

In thinking about transformation, the threshold between consciousness and surrender, I was reminded of a recent story. On a clear June day in 2025, fourteen-year-old Zane Wach summited Mount Whitney in the Sierra Nevada range of California—the highest peak in the continental United States—with his father by his side. As they descended, the thin air began to confuse his senses. Zane spoke of seeing Kermit the Frog, of snowmen in the rocks, of not knowing if he was awake or dreaming. "This isn't real," he said. "I don't think this is really happening." Moments later, he stepped off a 120-foot cliff and fell into silence. Incredibly, he survived—his body broken, his brain swelling, his breath kept alive by machines. Doctors believe he was suffering from high-altitude cerebral edema, a swelling of the brain that can cause hallucinations and confusion, especially in high-altitude, oxygen-poor places. But there was something hauntingly familiar about his words, something that felt less like illness and more like myth: a boy on the edge of the world, unsure whether he was dreaming or waking, speaking his last words from the threshold.[4]

Zane's story reminds us that the lines separating waking and dreaming and death, between consciousness and unconsciousness, are not as clean as we like to believe. Sleep—at least the approach we are exploring in this book—is not merely a biological reset; it's also a passage, a dissolution of boundaries. And so, too, is death. In Zane's moment of disorientation, what emerged was a profound image: a child, caught in a dream that felt more real than reality itself, stepping into the unknown. His fall was literal but also symbolic of how easily we slip between worlds.

Sleep is not just rest but a rehearsal for letting go, a gentle descent into mystery. What we call sleep, in its deepest forms, may not be so different from what lies beyond it. It isn't just where we shut off: It's where we show up. Each night, we're offered a mirror, a rehearsal, a return. In drifting away from the world, we return to something more essential: the part of us that watches, that remembers, that simply is. And in learning to meet sleep with awareness, we don't just sleep better; we awaken better. To our patterns. To our stories. To the selves we've hidden behind the busyness and noise. Sleep teaches us, quietly but persistently, that the boundary between waking and dreaming, between self and soul, is thinner than we think, gossamer, a barely-there veil. Maybe the real alchemy of sleep is this: By surrendering to sleep, we recover the parts of ourselves that never stopped dreaming. And in that quiet reunion, we remember who we were before the world told us to forget.

THE PLACE WE GO

In my early thirties, I nearly died. Somewhere between the brittle light of the Arizona desert and the familiar coastline of California, sleep took me. Not slowly, like the gentle fade we hope for in bed, but all at once. My body was awake until it wasn't. My hands slipped from the wheel, my eyes gave in, and for a moment, I no longer belonged to this world. What followed was not a crash in the cinematic sense but a subtle veer into a parallel realm: Consciousness folded inward, time dissolved. I was utterly gone.

And yet I returned.

I've never stopped thinking about that liminal space, that eerie overlap between sleep and death, between surrender and survival. If this book began in that space, it ends here, not in fear, but in awe. Because while sleep can mimic death, it also offers us something death cannot. A return. A second chance. A daily resurrection.

Sleep, like certain mythic narratives of descent, requires a journey downward. We fall, we cross thresholds, we shed the self. In ancient traditions, the sleeper journeys through night not unlike Orpheus in the underworld or Inanna descending into darkness. And yet, unlike mythic death, we do not need to be heroes to emerge. We only need to let go.

In a way, this book was my attempt to map a terrain no one else seemed to be charting, one where science holds hands with mystery, where case studies brush up against philosophy and meditation, where personal narrative weaves through it all. It is part memoir, part field guide, part love letter to a forgotten realm.

To sleep well is not simply to recharge. It is to remember who we are when no one is watching, when we are not performing or posting or persevering. It is to meet ourselves, stripped bare, in the dark. And be willing to return.

Tonight, when you close your eyes, you will practice a kind of dying. But more importantly, you will practice the art of return. You will enter the sacred laboratory of sleep, where the soul reshapes itself quietly and rhythmically. In the dark.

CONCLUSION

AS THE NIGHT SETTLES

As you reach the end of this book, I hope it's clear that sleep is not just something you have to do or wish you had more of but a living relationship that shapes every part of your life. Sleep is more than a nightly routine: It is a dynamic connection that deserves your attention, care, and growth—just like your friendships, your work, or your health.

In a world that so often asks us to sacrifice rest for productivity, reclaiming sleep as an act of self-respect and self-care is a quiet revolution. When you approach sleep holistically, tending to both the practical and the soulful, you create ripples that benefit your mind, body, and spirit. The way you prepare for sleep—how you wind down, how you set boundaries, and how you honor your need for rest—reflects the respect you show yourself in all areas of life.

Your relationship with sleep is always evolving. There is no single perfect way to rest. What works for you now may change as your life changes, and that's not a failure but a sign of growth. Flexibility, curiosity, and self-compassion are your greatest allies as you navigate the seasons of your sleep life. When challenges arise, whether it's a stretch of insomnia or a period of stress, remember that these are opportunities to listen, adapt, and deepen your understanding of what you need.

Sleep is a partner in your journey toward health and wholeness. It thrives on respect, patience, and forgiveness—forgiving yourself for the restless nights and celebrating the mornings when you wake restored. When you treat sleep as more than just a physical act, it becomes a practice of healing, alignment, and renewal.

As you lay your head down tonight, let gratitude guide you. Thank your body for carrying you through the day. Allow your mind to release what it no longer needs to hold. And remember: Sleep is not just a task, but a connection—a quiet space where you return to yourself, night after night. May you nurture this relationship, and may it nurture you in return.

AFTERWORD

THE FUTURE OF SLEEP

SLEEP MEDICINE IS STANDING AT THE EDGE OF SOMETHING unprecedented. While this book primarily focuses on transformative sleep practices rooted in longstanding psychological and spiritual traditions—an analog world, if you will—we are poised on the edge of a frontier rife with technology, rich with data. We are stepping into an era where the once opaque interiority of sleep is being made visible through hyper-personalized algorithms that tailor treatment to each sleeper's unique chronotype, genetic blueprint, and physiological signature. Technologies once confined to science fiction, such as AI-driven dream interpretation and the filming of dreams, are now breaching the edge of reality. We are witnessing the dawn of a sleep revolution, and I would be remiss to write a book about the alchemy of sleep and not acknowledge the dramatic transmutation that is imminent.

But as we race toward innovation, I offer a gentle caution: In our eagerness to decode and optimize, we must not lose touch with the ancient language of rest. Sleep is not merely a process to be measured or hacked; it is a rhythm, a ritual, a return. Our circadian rhythms evolved under the blue-black sky, in sync with tides, seasons, and stars. Personalized sleep medicine must honor the personal *and* the primordial. Dream recording may offer a mirror, but we should not forget the mystery.

The future of sleep medicine is dazzling and disorienting. But it will mean more if we remember where we came from: not from apps or analytics, but from dusk and stillness and silence. In looking ahead, let us not overwrite the past but carry it forward, encoded not just in data but in memory, biology, and myth.

PERSONALIZED SLEEP MEDICINE

In the past, and even now, treating sleep disorders such as insomnia, sleep apnea, or restless legs syndrome often felt like trial and error. A patient would try one treatment, then another, hoping something would eventually stick. As sleep specialists, we have all participated in this trial-and-error repertoire. But as our understanding of genetics, technology, and individual health grows, the future promises a shift toward precision. Personalized sleep medicine means using detailed information about your body—your genes, your metabolism, your environment—to create treatments that work specifically for you. Think of it as moving from a broad spotlight to a laser-focused beam.

One of the most exciting developments in personalized medicine is the role of genetics. Did you know that your genes can influence whether you're a night owl or a morning lark? Or whether you're prone to insomnia? In the future, a simple genetic test could help decode how your body processes sleep. For example, some individuals metabolize sleep medications quickly, while others may feel groggy for days after the same dose. By analyzing your DNA, doctors could prescribe the right medication in the right dose—or even suggest alternative treatment based on how your body works. For us sleep physicians, this would be invaluable data, preventing excessive grogginess in those for whom we prescribe hypnotics.

If you're wearing a smartwatch or a fitness tracker, you're already dipping your toes into personalized sleep medicine. Devices that measure sleep stages, heart rate, and oxygen levels are becoming more sophisticated every year. In the future, these gadgets could do much more than track your sleep; they could predict problems before they start. Imagine a wearable device that alerts you to early signs of sleep apnea before you even notice the telltale signs such as snoring, cessation of breathing, and so forth. Or one that adjusts the temperature of your bedroom based on your body's ideal sleep environment. The data these devices collect will feed directly into your personalized treatment plan that we as sleep specialists can then design.

For some, treatment might involve cutting-edge therapies such as neurostimulation, where gentle electrical impulses help regulate brain activity during sleep. For others, it could mean targeted behavioral strategies or even microbiome adjustments—because, yes, the bacteria in your gut might play a role in how well you sleep. Medication will also look different. Instead of standard sleep aids, we might receive a drug designed specifically for our genetic makeup, reducing side effects and improving efficacy.

Here's where it gets even more futuristic. Artificial intelligence is already changing how we diagnose and treat diseases, and sleep medicine is no exception. AI could analyze your sleep patterns, medical history, and lifestyle factors to create a dynamic, evolving treatment plan. Picture this: You wake up, and your sleep app analyzes your night's data. It notices whether you had fragmented sleep and suggests a specific breathing exercise or a minor dietary tweak for the day. Over time, the system learns what works for you, becoming smarter and more precise with every interaction.

The future of sleep gadgets is heading straight into the realm of personalized, responsive environments, too: smart bedrooms that know *you*. Imagine a system that detects your ideal sleeping temperature and quietly adjusts the thermostat on your side, while also syncing with circadian lighting tuned to your biology—cooler, blue tones in the morning for the teenager who cannot wake up before 9:00 a.m. and warmer, dimmer light at night for the average person winding down after a long day. In this future, your home could subtly manipulate light exposure throughout the day to keep your internal clock on track, gradually dimming in the evening without you even touching a switch. Add in soundscapes that adjust to stress levels or phase out street noise, and you've got an environment that acts like a sleep concierge. Picture a household where everyone's bedroom lighting, temperature, and ambiance are individually tuned to optimize their sleep cycles: no more "one thermostat fits all." It's like having a sleep lab built into your home but way cozier. These small changes could impact your sleep, and health, dramatically.

Despite all this amazing technology, one thing remains constant: the importance of the doctor-patient relationship. Personalized sleep medicine doesn't mean replacing doctors with machines. Instead, it enhances the tools that we doctors possess to provide better care. Your doctor might sit down with a detailed profile of your sleep health, complete with genetic insights, wearable data, and AI-driven recommendations. Together, you'll craft a plan that not only improves your sleep but also fits seamlessly into your life.

The future of personalized sleep medicine, as I routinely tell my patients, is essentially about empowerment. It's about giving you the tools and knowledge to take control of your sleep health. Instead of feeling frustrated or stuck, you'll have a roadmap tailored just for you. So, whether you're someone who struggles to fall asleep, wakes up too often, or just wants to optimize your rest, the future promises treatments that are as unique and dynamic as you are. Sleep, once a mystery, will become a science deeply personal to each of us. But remember, don't rely solely on technology; use it to augment your sleep using the methods that I presented throughout this book.

A philosophical concept may serve as a warning here to the technologies that we're overusing for sleep, as I repeatedly tell my patients. The philosopher Robert Pfaller coined the term *interpassivity* to describe the paradoxical condition in which we outsource enjoyment, belief, or even experience itself to another agent—human or nonhuman—who acts in our stead.[1] The philosopher Slavoi Žižek expanded on the idea, showing how cultural forms "believe" or "enjoy" on our behalf: the sitcom laugh track that chuckles for us, the ritual that sustains belief when we are cynics.[2] Interpassivity is, in short, the delegation of our inner life to an external proxy.

Nowhere is this more vivid than in modern sleep culture. We wear rings and watches that do the "sleeping" for us, telling us whether we truly rested, even when our bodies already know. We hand our serenity over to meditation apps that whisper bedtime stories or to pills that sleep in our place. Dream journals and AI interpreters metabolize the unconscious before we ever confront it. These devices and rituals enact what Pfaller warned: a cultural drift in which belief and experience are no longer ours but are sustained elsewhere on our behalf. Sleep itself becomes interpassive: We slumber less in our own bodies and more through our proxies, allowing technology, ritual, or pharmacology to carry the burden—and enjoyment—of rest.

But why do we delegate enjoyment when it's supposed to make us feel good? Pfaller reminds us that enjoyment today is not simply an option but an obligation. We are told, indeed urged, to relax, to savor, to rest well, to sleep eight hours or more—as if pleasure were another item on the to-do list. That pressure can be paralyzing, as I so often tell my patients. Interpassivity offers false relief: We let devices, rituals, or substances "enjoy" for us, carrying the weight of expectation so we don't have to. We delegate not because we do not value enjoyment or our sleep but because the demand to enjoy, to rest well, to sleep well, has itself become exhausting.

As we cross into this new frontier, may we remember that true rest is not something that can be fully outsourced or measured but something we experience in the quiet, unquantifiable spaces within ourselves. The future of sleep will be richest when it honors both our capacity for innovation and our need for mystery, allowing us to move forward without losing touch with the ancient wisdom that has always guided us home to rest.

FILMING THE UNCONSCIOUS

Dr. Evelyn Carter adjusted the EEG electrodes on the young volunteer's scalp, her fingers moving with the precision of years spent navigating the fragile bridge between sleep and wakefulness. Across the dimly lit lab, screens flickered with colorful waves of neural activity: electrical echoes of a mind slipping into REM sleep, into dreams, into the unknown.

"This is it," she murmured. "Tonight, we catch a dream."

Beside her, Dr. Marcus Patel tapped furiously on his keyboard, calibrating the fMRI scanner. "I don't know if we're ready to call it 'catching' just yet," he said. "More like . . . reconstructing a ghost from static."

The Dream Recording Project—an ambitious endeavor led by a coalition of neuroscientists, AI engineers, neurologists (including me), and dream researchers such as Daniel Oldis, who helms the project—had been progressing for years, inching closer to what had been science fiction: recording and visualizing dreams. It was no longer just a fantasy of William Gibson's cyberpunk novels. With rapid advancements in neuroimaging, machine learning, and brain-computer interfaces, the team was on the verge of translating raw brain signals into moving images.

Tonight's experiment was simple in theory, maddeningly complex in execution. A volunteer—Brian, a college student at Stanford known for his vivid and unusual dreams—would fall asleep while connected to an EEG, fMRI, and an array of high-density electrodes. As he dreamed, artificial intelligence would analyze his brain activity in real-time, comparing it against massive databases of previously mapped neural imagery. The goal? To reconstruct, with some degree of clarity, the dream playing out behind Brian's closed eyelids.

Marcus leaned back, exhaling sharply. "I still don't understand how Oldis and his team got their dream speech model to work. That's some impressive shit."

Evelyn smirked. "You just don't like that language processing has outpaced our visual model."

"Because visuals are the holy grail," Marcus said, shaking his head. "Think about it. If we can map neural firing patterns to images, we're literally making dreams visible. That's . . ." He hesitated, searching for a word that fit. "That's breaking the final barrier between mind and machine."

Evelyn didn't argue. She understood his frustration. Oldis and his colleagues had made incredible progress in decoding dream speech—translating imagined words and phrases into actual text using brainwave activity. But the full cinematic dreamscape, composed of the landscape, faces, and impossible architecture, remained elusive. They could generate rough approximations from fMRI data, but they were still a long way from replaying a dream with Hollywood clarity and production design.

A soft beep interrupted her thoughts.

Brian's heart rate became more variable, more erratic. His eyes darted back and forth under closed eyelids. The classic sign of REM sleep.

"He's in," Evelyn whispered.

The software whirred to life, running predictive models at lightning speed. The AI began interpreting patterns, translating Brian's flickering neuronal signals into fragmented images. At first, it was static, then came abstract shapes, flashes of color, shadow.

Then, a hazy figure.

"Wait . . . are we seeing this?" Marcus whispered.

The screen showed a blurry approximation of a person, who was distorted, almost like an old VHS recording playing a half-erased scene. The AI struggled, reshaping the form every few seconds, as if uncertain what it was seeing.

Evelyn's heart pounded. "Enhance the contrast," she said.

Marcus adjusted the parameters. The image sharpened slightly. The outline of a woman, long hair, a faint glow behind her like a gossamer shadow.

Brian stirred in his sleep. His lips moved imperceptibly. The speech model activated, filtering neural signals into readable text. A garbled message appeared on the screen:

"She was here before . . . I remember . . . the blue door."

Evelyn's skin prickled.

Marcus glanced at her. "Do we wake him?"

"No," she said.

As Evelyn and Marcus watched the fragmented images flicker on the screen, they knew they were standing at the edge of something groundbreaking, yet still incomplete. The technology was in its infancy, producing hazy glimpses rather than full cinematic dreams, but with rapid advances in AI and neuroimaging, the day when dreams could be truly "filmed" no longer seemed like science fiction. It was just a matter of time.

As the scene above depicts, we're not quite at the level of "filming" dreams right now, but we're closer than ever to decoding them. Scientists, including Daniel Oldis and research teams in Japan and the United States, have already used fMRI and AI models to reconstruct basic images from brain activity.[3] These images are blurry, impressionistic shapes, kind of like an old, static-filled TV screen. They've even made progress in translating dream speech: the words we "say" in our minds while dreaming. The challenge is that dreams are wildly complex, blending memory, imagination, and emotion in a way that doesn't follow strict visual rules. But with the rapid evolution of AI, neuroimaging, and brain-computer interfaces, many believe we could see rudimentary dream playback within the next ten to twenty years. Nothing Hollywood-ready or Oscars-worthy, but enough to glimpse the hidden world of our sleeping minds.

The fundamental challenge of filming a dream is that dreaming is a subjective experience: It is trapped within the sleeper's mind. Unlike external stimuli that can be directly observed, dreams exist in the private theater of the brain. To unlock them, scientists must rely on indirect measures: brain activity, eye movements, and even muscle twitches.

The key player in this field is functional magnetic resonance imaging (fMRI), which detects changes in blood flow to different brain regions, and electroencephalography (EEG), which records electrical activity. These tools allow researchers to track which areas of the brain light up during dreaming, offering clues about the content of dreams. But how do we translate those signals into something recognizable, something we could watch?

One of the most groundbreaking studies on dream decoding was conducted by the Japanese neuroscientist Yukiyasu Kamitani and his team at Kyoto University.[4] Their approach was simple yet ingenious. First, participants were shown thousands of images while inside an fMRI scanner. By analyzing which brain regions responded to different images, researchers created a "dictionary" of how the brain represents visual experiences. Next, participants took a nap inside the scanner. Every time the EEG detected that they had entered early dream stages, researchers woke them up and asked what they had been dreaming about. This was repeated many times, with the AI linking reported dream content to corresponding brain activity. Finally, the AI used this information to make predictions: Based on the brain activity alone, could it guess what the person was dreaming about? The results were astonishing. If a person dreamed of a cat, the AI produced a blurry but recognizable image of a cat. If the dream featured buildings, the AI generated a rough sketch of architectural structures. While not perfect, it was a first glimpse into the possibility of visualizing dreams.

The biggest hurdle in reconstructing dreams is their unpredictable nature. Unlike waking perception, which follows external stimuli, dreams emerge from a complex interplay of memory, emotion, and subconscious associations. The same neural patterns that correspond to a "dog" while awake might represent something entirely different in a dream. Another challenge is that dreams are often non-static, that is, they morph, shift, defy logical structure. How do you film something that doesn't follow a linear storyline? Some researchers are now exploring whether AI can reconstruct not just static dream images but entire sequences, piecing together how a dream unfolds over time.

While we're still far from pressing "record" on our dreams, the field is advancing rapidly. Some researchers predict that within a few decades, we may have technology capable of providing detailed visual reconstructions of our dreams. This could revolutionize everything from dream analysis in therapy to new forms of storytelling. Imagine filmmakers literally pulling ideas straight from their dreams and producing an avant-garde production that we can only imagine. A seismic shift in the film industry would occur, of a magnitude that would likely leave us speechless and alter the economic landscape of Hollywood.

But this also raises ethical questions and issues: Should our dreams remain private, or could future technology allow them to be involuntarily accessed and be commoditized for mass consumption? At what point does a dream stop being personal and start being property? Whose dreams get shared, and who decides? Using the dreams of celebrities might draw crowds, but it raises the questions of exploitation and consent. And what about "ordinary" people—do their dreams get sidelined, or worse, edited for drama? If we could relive our dreams, would we spend too much time escaping into them and have difficulty separating reality from fiction? In an age of deepfakes and digital surveillance, translating dreams into entertainment could blur lines we haven't even drawn yet. For now, though, the dream remains just out of focus. But stay tuned and keep watching, because the signal is getting clearer, sharper, and crisper.

ACKNOWLEDGMENTS

TO MY AGENT, LINDA KONNER—THANK YOU FOR BELIEVING IN this strange, genre-defying project from the beginning and championing it with such heart. Your unwavering support, strategic brilliance, and instinct for where this book needed to go have made all the difference.

To my editor, the fearless Jenn Brown—immense thanks. I'm deeply grateful for your sharp editorial eye and deep understanding of sleep that helped shape this book into something more lucid than I ever imagined. Your ability to see both the structure and soul of a manuscript made this a far richer and more coherent work than it had any right to be. I'm also extremely grateful for your encouragement and being there amid the storm. Truly.

To the entire team at Shambhala Publications, especially Sara Bercholz, Ivan Bercholz, and Nikko Odiseos—thank you for welcoming this book into your visionary catalogue. Your commitment to ideas that stretch across science, spirit, and the soul has long inspired me, and I'm honored to be part of your literary lineage.

To my good friend and former professor, Rey Chow—your brilliance continues to stretch my thinking and inspire how I write. You taught me that theory can be poetic and that language, like identity, is always more layered than it seems. In the past year, you have also taught me to weather the storm without losing sight of the dry terrain just ahead. I'm forever indebted to you.

I owe deep thanks to Stephen Brooks, Christian Guilleminault, Rafael Pelayo, and Anstella Robinson (and my fellow colleagues Gwynne Church and Michael Zupancic) at the Stanford Sleep Disorders Clinic, whose mentorship and camaraderie brought clarity, depth, and wonder to my understanding of sleep. They showed me that sleep is not merely studied: It is listened to.

My sincere thanks go to the sleep physicians, staff, and sleep technicians at the Hoag Voltmer Sleep Center—particularly Dr. Gozzo, Dr. Puango, and Miki Ohata—who created an environment of generosity and understanding that allowed me the time to work through ideas, fill countless notebooks, and write. Their quiet support is woven throughout these pages.

An enormous thanks to Dr. Andrew Weil, Dr. Adam Gavsie, and everyone at the Andrew Weil Center for Integrative Medicine for orienting me to a wider, richer view of integrative care. I learned so much from you all. You made even the most ordinary moments feel spacious, generous, and quietly extraordinary.

To my friends and family, as always, thank you for the patience, the encouragement, and the love. There are too many to name here, but you all know who you are and how much I care for each of you. My love knows no bounds for you.

And, not least, an immense thanks to my twin sister, Pooneh, and to my parents, who have been instrumental in all things, seen and unseen. No words fully capture what your presence and support have meant to me.

This book was born from a desire to write what I hadn't seen written, a space where neuroscience, metaphysics, and spirituality could share a bed alongside fragments of my own story. To every reader who carried this book to their bedside: Thank you for letting my words rest with you.

APPENDIX A

SLEEP HYGIENE CHECKLIST

SLEEP HYGIENE IS A COLLECTION OF PRACTICES AND HABITS that support consistent, restorative sleep. Practicing good sleep hygiene means creating routines and surroundings that signal to your body that it's time to wind down. Think of it as laying the foundation for better sleep. Throughout this book, I've covered many aspects of sleep hygiene: such as the importance of temperature, lighting, food choices, and mindset. I've pulled together the most important ones here for easy reference. This list isn't about perfection; it's about developing habits that support restful sleep. Start with a few changes and build from there—over time, you'll create an environment and mindset where good sleep feels natural. Any bedtime ritual you create to help you sleep (see appendix B) will be much more effective when built on these healthy foundations. By making these practices part of your daily life, you'll find your sleep—and your overall well-being—begin to improve.

- *Create your sleep sanctuary.* Keep your bedroom quiet, dark, and cool (60–67°F/16–19°C). Use blackout curtains or an eye mask and minimize light from electronics—move your phone out of reach or turn it face down. Even small lights can disrupt sleep. Declutter your space: A tidy room calms the mind and reduces mental load.
- *Stick to a sleep schedule.* Go to bed and wake up at the same times every day, even on weekends. This helps regulate your internal clock. If you struggle with this, reward yourself for consistency—maybe with a favorite morning ritual. Avoid hitting snooze, as it disrupts your natural sleep cycle and can leave you groggy.
- *Wind down before bed.* Begin slowing down about two hours before sleep. Dim the lights and turn off screens at least an hour before bed to avoid blue light and mental stimulation. Instead, read a physical book, meditate, journal, or take a warm bath. As your body cools down after the bath, it can help signal to your brain that it's time for sleep. Avoid stressful activities and all social media, which are designed to keep you alert and engaged.
- *Watch what you eat and drink.* Limit caffeine after midafternoon and avoid heavy or spicy meals close to bedtime. Alcohol may make you sleepy at first but disrupts deep sleep later. If you drink, keep it light and finish at least three hours before bed. Hydrate early but avoid lots of fluids right before sleep to minimize nighttime awakenings.
- *Move your body.* Exercise regularly, but not too close to bedtime. Gentle stretching or yoga in the evening can help relax your body and mind.
- *Keep naps short and early.* If you nap, keep it under thirty minutes and avoid late-day naps to prevent interference with nighttime sleep.

- *Calm your mind.* Practice deep breathing, mindfulness, or guided imagery anytime during the day. If your mind is racing, jot down your thoughts to "park" them. Visualize calming scenes or recall positive memories to shift your focus away from worries.
- *Restrict non-sleep time in bed.* If you spend much more time in bed than you're actually sleeping, try limiting your time in bed to match your actual sleep time. As your sleep becomes more efficient, you can gradually increase your time in bed. If you can't sleep after twenty minutes, get up and do something relaxing in low light. Avoid checking the time, which only increases anxiety.
- *Limit bed activities.* Reserve your bed primarily for sleep, intimacy, and low-light reading or journaling. If you can't sleep, leave the bedroom and return only when you feel sleepy. This helps your brain associate the bed with rest, not wakefulness.
- *Change your attitude about sleep and wakefulness.* Reframing your relationship to sleep—and to the challenges that come with it—means approaching both rest and wakefulness with curiosity and acceptance rather than frustration or fear. By shifting your mindset, you create space for greater ease, allowing sleep to become a supportive, restorative part of your life rather than a nightly struggle.

APPENDIX B

CREATING YOUR OWN BEDTIME RITUAL

SOME NIGHTS, LIKE EVERYONE ELSE, MY BRAIN WON'T SHUT OFF. It loops through everything I didn't do, everything I said wrong, everything that I still must hold together. Work stress, too much time online, and maybe a late dinner or too much caffeine can sometimes leave me "twired"—tired but wired.

What helps most is when I stop pretending that I'm supposed to be calm. I sit on the edge of my bed and name three things I'm grateful for. I attempt to anchor myself to something that won't unravel. Sometimes it's just: "I'm still here. I'm not living on the street. I still have breath. I get another shot tomorrow." Then I lie down and press my hand to my chest—not for the sake of mindfulness, but to remind myself that I'm real, that I made it through the day, that I have loved ones. This has become my occasional ritual. It's messy, kind of strange, but it works. And slowly, sleep comes. Not because I force it, but because I finally stop fighting. I surrender. It sometimes feels like a kind of forgiveness.

A consistent bedtime routine serves as a signal to the brain that it's time to unwind. Preparation is important, but not to the point of overthinking—sleep isn't a switch you flip, but a gentle dimming of the lights that happens throughout your day. When you combine the practicalities of what are commonly called "sleep hygiene" with psychological and spiritual elements, you begin to reorient your life in a way that honors the importance of sleep to the very core of your body, mind, and spirit. You begin to treat sleep as a sacred experience.

An effective bedtime sleep ritual is more than a series of steps: It's a transformative practice that bridges science and spirituality bringing body, mind, and spirit into harmony and connecting you to your deeper self. By blending evidence-based strategies with grounding rituals, you can create a bedtime routine that not only improves sleep but also fosters a more balanced outlook on life. What you create will look different from my funny ritual and from everyone else's, but that's the beauty of it. By discovering what works for you, you drop into deeper relationship with yourself, and that will have echoes that reverberate well beyond your relationship with sleep.

A bedtime ritual is a gift you give yourself—a way to honor your need for rest and renewal. A ritual contains certain components, but it can be customized to your needs, and it can change, evolving with your life. Over time, this nightly practice can become not just a way to fall asleep but a way to come home to yourself, again and again. Remember, consistency is more important than perfection, so stick with it. Over time, you're sure to notice changes.

Here is a general outline for creating a bedtime ritual, followed by details for each step. You don't have to choose something from every category. Pick what calls to you and let your ritual evolve from there.

- Prepare your environment, making your space cool, dark, and quiet.
- Choose grounding practices for the body.
- Add calming practices for the mind.
- Enjoy connection and touch with another or a pet—or some self-touch.
- Practice gratitude.
- Set an intention.
- Include a spiritual or contemplative element.

- ***Ground your body.*** Our bodies are the stage on which sleep's nightly drama unfolds. Gentle movement—yoga, stretching, or a warm bath—can signal to your nervous system that it's time to unwind. Essential oils, such as lavender, and the simple comfort of soft pajamas or a heavy blanket help anchor you in the present moment. As you move through your ritual, let each sensation remind you: It's safe to let go.
- ***Calm your mind.*** So many of us fight sleep, clinging to our thoughts like wreckage in a storm, afraid that if we surrender, we'll lose something vital. But sleep waits for us like a forgiving lover we keep abandoning. Mindfulness meditation, journaling, breathwork, or reading poetry or other quieting material can help you loosen your grip on the day. Try writing down what brought you peace, not just what went wrong. Let your mind settle, like silt in a pond, until the water is clear again.
- ***Touch and connection.*** Connection soothes the heart. You may try affectionate touch with a loved one, a cuddle with a pet, or a mindful gesture of self-compassion. Sleep is a time when we can lay down our armor and be held—by another or by ourselves.

- *Practice gratitude.* Gratitude is a gentle but profound reorientation of the heart. The practice of noticing and appreciating what's positive in your life, gratitude can be a powerful way to improve sleep. By focusing on what went well, even small things, you shift your attention away from stress and anxiety, creating a sense of safety and calm. Research shows that keeping a gratitude journal before bed helps people sleep better and longer, as it reframes the day in a positive light and eases mental burdens. Each night, write down three specific things you're grateful for and why they mattered to you. If nothing joyful comes to mind, note what could have gone wrong but didn't. Over time, this simple practice can help replace worry with a more peaceful mindset.[1]
- *Set an intention.* Sleep is a threshold, a crossing. Setting an intention—whether it's for rest, healing, or simply to let go—can transform your experience. Setting intentions means creating a purposeful mindset for both sleep and, possibly, for the following day. By focusing your mind on a calming intention—such as "I am ready to let go of today and embrace rest"—you help ease the shift from wakefulness to sleep. This practice can also help you if you tend to wake up into negativity, immediately anticipating the difficulties of the day. You can write down an intention, such as "Today, I will approach challenges with calm and clarity," and have it ready by your bedside to read in the morning.
- *Tap into spirit.* Sleep is also a spiritual act. In the quiet hours, we are closest to our own depths. Prayer, meditation, or reading a spiritual text can invite a sense of the sacred into your ritual. You may also try visualizations, such as imagining yourself surrounded by soothing light or having a dialogue with a guide, a loved one who has passed, or other spirit connection.

SAMPLE BEDTIME RITUALS

Short Ritual (10 Minutes)

Dim the lights, put your phone away, tidy your bedside.

Write down three things you're grateful for.

Do two to three minutes of gentle stretching or deep breathing.

Set a simple intention for rest.

Visualize a calming scene or offer a brief affirmation.

Longer Ritual (20–30 Minutes)

Adjust lighting, light a candle, ensure your room is cool and quiet.

Take a warm bath or shower with calming essential oils.

Spend five to ten minutes journaling about your day, focusing on what went well.

Write or speak three things you're grateful for.

Read an affirmation or meditate for a few minutes.

Share a hug, cuddle a pet, or place a hand on your heart.

Extended Ritual (45–60 Minutes)

Declutter your room, set the temperature, use blackout curtains, and play soft music.

Do ten minutes of gentle yoga or stretching, followed by a warm bath with lavender oil.

Do ten minutes of mindful reading (inspirational or spiritual text).

Reflect on the day in a journal, focusing on peace and gratitude.

Write an intention for your sleep or dreams.

Meditate or visualize a peaceful place.

Connect with a loved one or practice self-compassion.

Blow out a candle or turn off the lights, and take a few deep breaths as you settle in.

RITUALS FOR PARENTS, SHIFT WORKERS, AND TRAVELERS

Rituals can sometimes be easier to create in a life that has some routine and predictability. As a physician who has often worked crazy hours, I know that not all of us have lives that follow predictable schedules. Here are some ways that parents, shift workers, and those who travel frequently can bring some bedtime rituals into their lives.

For parents, a bedtime ritual can become a meaningful family tradition. Try gathering everyone for a brief gratitude circle, where each person shares something positive from their day. Follow this with a calming bedtime story and gentle music to help children unwind. After the kids are asleep, take a few moments for your own self-care practice, whether that's reading, stretching, or simply taking a few deep breaths to mark the transition into your own rest.

Shift workers face unique challenges when it comes to sleep, but a consistent pre-sleep routine can make a significant difference—even if your "night" falls during daylight hours. Use blackout curtains to block out sunlight and create a dark, restful environment. White noise can help mask daytime sounds, making it easier to drift off. Try to follow the same wind-down steps before each sleep period, such as dimming lights, reading, or practicing relaxation techniques to signal to your body that it's time for rest, regardless of what the time on the clock says.

For travelers, maintaining a sense of continuity and comfort is key to restful sleep away from home. Pack an eye mask to block out unfamiliar light and bring along a calming tea or scent to create a familiar, soothing atmosphere. Before bed, repeat a favorite affirmation or visualization that helps you feel grounded and safe. These small rituals can help your mind and body relax, no matter where you are. And revisit the instructions in chapter 9, "Harnessing the Power of Light and Dark," to work with your circadian rhythm.

SLEEP AS SACRED SELF-CARE

I hope by now you have come to see sleep not just as a nightly requirement but as a profound act of self-care and reconnection. When you approach sleep as something sacred—something that deserves your attention, preparation, and even reverence—you begin to change your relationship not only with rest but with yourself. The science and the soul of sleep are not at odds; together, they offer a path toward healing, resilience, and a deeper sense of belonging in your own life.

Integrating these practices may not always be seamless. There will be nights when your mind races, when routines are disrupted, or when sleep feels far away. But each time you return to your ritual, no matter how simple or imperfect, you are making a quiet commitment to your own well-being. Over time, these small acts of care accumulate, gently reshaping your nights and your days.

May you find, in the quiet space between wakefulness and sleep, a place to lay down your burdens and remember what is most essential. May your rituals—however ordinary or unusual—become a source of comfort, healing, and discovery. And may you come to trust that, in tending to your sleep, you are tending to every part of your life.

NOTES

Introduction

1. Christopher P. Landrigan, Jeffrey M. Rothschild, John W. Cronin, Rainu Kaushal, Elisabeth Burdick, Joel T. Katz et al., "Effect of Reducing Interns' Work Hours on Serious Medical Errors in Intensive Care Units," *New England Journal of Medicine* 351, no. 18 (October 28, 2004): 1838–48, https://doi.org/10.1056/nejmoa041406.
2. Marco Hafner, Martin Stepanek, Jirka Taylor, Wendy M. Troxel, and Christian Van Stolk, "Why Sleep Matters—the Economic Costs of Insufficient Sleep: A Cross-Country Comparative Analysis," RAND, November 30, 2016, https://www.rand.org/pubs/research_reports/RR1791.html.
3. Maurice Blanchot, *The Space of Literature* (University of Nebraska Press, 1982).
4. Pema Chödrön, *How We Live Is How We Die* (Shambhala Publications, 2022).
5. Octavia F. Raheem, *Rest Is Sacred: Reclaiming Our Brilliance Through the Practice of Stillness* (Shambhala Publications, 2024).

1. Sleep Is Your Body's Superpower

1. A. Rechtschaffen, "The Control of Sleep," in *Human Behavior and Its Control*, ed. William Hunt (Schenkman Publishing, 1971).
2. Matthew Walker, *Why We Sleep: Unlocking the Power of Sleep and Dreams* (Scribner, 2018), 72–76.
3. A. Roger Ekirch, *At Day's Close: Night in Times Past* (W. W. Norton & Company, 2006).
4. Frederick L. Coolidge, *Evolutionary Neuropsychology: An Introduction to the Evolution of the Structures and Functions of the Human Brain* (Oxford University Press, 2020).

5. H. H. the Fourteenth Dalai Lama, *Where Buddhism Meets Neuroscience: Conversations with the Dalai Lama on the Spiritual and Scientific Views of Our Minds* (Shambhala Publications, 2018), 98.
6. Denise J. Cai, Sarnoff A. Mednik, Elizabeth M. Harrison, Jennifer C. Kanady, and Sara C. Mednik, "REM, Not Incubation, Improves Creativity by Priming Associative Networks," *Proceedings of the National Academy of Sciences* 106, no. 25 (June 9, 2009): 10130–34, https://doi.org/10.1073/pnas.0900271106.
7. Matthew P. Walker and Els Van Der Helm, "Overnight Therapy? The Role of Sleep in Emotional Brain Processing," *Psychological Bulletin* 135, no. 5 (January 1, 2009): 731–48, https://doi.org/10.1037/a0016570.
8. Seung-Schik Yoo, Ninad Gujar, Peter Hu, Ferenc A. Jolesz, and Matthew P. Walker, "The Human Emotional Brain Without Sleep—a Prefrontal Amygdala Disconnect," *Current Biology* 17, no. 20 (October 1, 2007): R877–78, https://doi.org/10.1016/j.cub.2007.08.007.
9. Michel Jouvet, "Locus coeruleus et sommeil paradoxal," *Comptes rendus des séances de la Société de biologie et de ses filiales* 159 (1965): 895–99.
10. Coolidge, *Evolutionary Neuropsychology*, 187.
11. Walker, *Why We Sleep*, 110–11.
12. Coolidge, *Evolutionary Neuropsychology*, 190.
13. Walker, *Why We Sleep*, 128–31.
14. Walker, *Why We Sleep*, 131.
15. Aric A. Prather, Martica Hall, Jacqueline M. Fury, Diana C. Ross, Matthew F. Muldoon, Sheldon Cohen et al., "Sleep and Antibody Response to Hepatitis B Vaccination," *Sleep* 35, no. 8 (August 1, 2012): 1063–69, https://doi.org/10.5665/sleep.1990.
16. Karine Spiegel, John F. Sheridan, and Eve Van Cauter, "Effect of Sleep Deprivation on Response to Immunizaton," *JAMA* 288, no. 12 (September 25, 2002): 1471-a, https://doi.org/10.1001/jama.288.12.1471-a.
17. Sheldon Cohen, William J. Doyle, Cuneyt M. Alper, Denise Janicki-Deverts, and Ronald B. Turner, "Sleep Habits and Susceptibility to the Common Cold," *Archives of Internal Medicine* 169, no. 1 (January 12, 2009): 62, https://doi.org/10.1001/archinternmed.2008.505.
18. Raheem, *Rest Is Sacred*, 10.

2. How Sleep Unlocks Your Brain's Potential

1. Seung-Schik Yoo, Ninad Gujar, Peter Hu, Ferenc A. Jolesz, and Matthew P. Walker, "The Human Emotional Brain Without Sleep—a Prefrontal Amygdala Disconnect," *Current Biology* 17, no. 20 (October 1, 2007): R877–78, https://doi.org/10.1016/j.cub.2007.08.007.

2. Jared D. Minkel, S. Banks, O. Htaik, M. C. Moreta, C. W. Jones, E. L. McGlinchey et al., "Sleep Deprivation and Stressors: Evidence for Elevated Negative Affect in Response to Mild Stressors When Sleep Deprived," *Emotion* 12, no. 5 (January 1, 2012): 1015–20, https://doi.org/10.1037/a0026871.
3. Els Van Der Helm, Ninad Gujar, and Matthew P. Walker, "Sleep Deprivation Impairs the Accurate Recognition of Human Emotions," *Sleep* 33, no. 3 (March 1, 2010): 335–42, https://doi.org/10.1093/sleep/33.3.335.

3. Common Sleep Disorders

1. Jiongjiong Wang, Marc Korczykowski, Hengyi Rao, Yong Fan, John Pluta, Ruben C. Gur et al., "Gender Difference in Neural Response to Psychological Stress," *Social Cognitive and Affective Neuroscience* 2, no. 3 (May 24, 2007): 227–39, https://doi.org/10.1093/scan/nsm018.
2. Andrew Weil, *Mind Over Meds: Know When Drugs Are Necessary, When Alternatives Are Better, and When to Let Your Body Heal on Its Own* (Little, Brown, 2017), 91.
3. Noriko Shinjyo, Guy Waddell, and Julia Green, "Valerian Root in Treating Sleep Problems and Associated Disorders—A Systematic Review and Meta-Analysis," *Journal of Evidence-Based Integrative Medicine* 25 (January 1, 2020): 2515690X2096732, https://doi.org/10.1177/2515690x20967323.
4. Mohsen Adib-Hajbaghery and Seyedeh Nesa Mousavi, "The Effects of Chamomile Extract on Sleep Quality Among Elderly People: A Clinical Trial," *Complementary Therapies in Medicine* 35 (October 14, 2017): 109–14, https://doi.org/10.1016/j.ctim.2017.09.010.
5. A. Ngan and R. Conduit, "A Double-Blind, Placebo-Controlled Investigation of the Effects of Passiflora Incarnata (Passionflower) Herbal Tea on Subjective Sleep Quality," *Phytotherapy Research* 25, no. 8 (February 3, 2011): 1153–59, https://doi.org/10.1002/ptr.3400.
6. Angela Smith Lillehei, Linda L. Halcon, Kay Savik, Reilly Reis, "Effect of Inhaled Lavender and Sleep Hygiene on Self-Reported Sleep Issues: A Randomized Controlled Trial," *The Journal of Alternative and Complementary Medicine* 21, no. 7 (July 1, 2015): 430–38, https://doi.org/10.1089/acm.2014.0327.
7. Deepak Langade, Vaishali Thakare, Subodh Kanchi, and Sunil Kelgane, "Clinical Evaluation of the Pharmacological Impact of Ashwagandha Root Extract on Sleep in Healthy Volunteers and Insomnia Patients: A Double-Blind, Randomized, Parallel-Group, Placebo-Controlled Study," *Journal of Ethnopharmacology* 264 (August 17, 2020): 113276, https://doi.org/10.1016/j.jep.2020.113276.

8. Julien Cases, Alvin Ibarra, Nicolas Feuillere, Marc Roller, and Samir Sukkar, "Pilot Trial of Melissa Officinalis L. Leaf Extract in the Treatment of Volunteers Suffering from Mild-to-Moderate Anxiety Disorders and Sleep Disturbances," *Mediterranean Journal of Nutrition and Metabolism* 4, no. 3 (December 16, 2010): 211–18, https://doi.org/10.1007/s12349-010-0045-4.
9. Wataru Yamadera, Kentaro Inagawa, Shintaro Chiba, Makoto Bannai, Michio Takahashi, and Kazuhiko Nakayama, "Glycine Ingestion Improves Subjective Sleep Quality in Human Volunteers, Correlating with Polysomnographic Changes," *Sleep and Biological Rhythms* 5, no. 2 (March 27, 2007): 126–31, https://doi.org/10.1111/j.1479-8425.2007.00262.x.
10. Chogyal Namkhai Norbu and Jamgon Mipham, *Buddhist Dream Yoga: Dzogchen and the Practice of Natural Light* (Shambhala Publications, 2025), 18.
11. Yi Yu, Xinju Li, Zheng Zhu, Yingdong Wang, Qiang Xi, Jiwen Qiu et al., "Acupuncture for Chronic Insomnia Disorder: A Systematic Review with Meta-Analysis and Trial Sequential Analysis," *Frontiers in Neurology* 16 (April 30, 2025): 1541276, https://doi.org/10.3389/fneur.2025.1541276.
12. David S. Black, Gillian A. O'Reilly, Richard Omstead, Elizabeth C. Breen, and Michael R. Irwin, "Mindfulness Meditation and Improvement in Sleep Quality and Daytime Impairment Among Older Adults with Sleep Disturbances," *JAMA Internal Medicine* 175, no. 4 (February 16, 2015): 494, https://doi.org/10.1001/jamainternmed.2014.8081.
13. Bodil Ekholm, Stefan Spulber, and Mats Adler, "A Randomized Controlled Study of Weighted Chain Blankets for Insomnia in Psychiatric Disorders," *Journal of Clinical Sleep Medicine* 16, no. 9 (June 15, 2020): 1567–77, https://doi.org/10.5664/jcsm.8636.
14. Maren J. Cordi, Angelika A. Schlarb, and Björn Rasch, "Deepening Sleep by Hypnotic Suggestion," *Sleep* 37, no. 6 (May 30, 2014): 1143–52, https://doi.org/10.5665/sleep.3778.
15. Fang Wang, Othelia Eun-Kyound Lee, Fan Feng, Michael V. Vitiello, Weidong Wang, Herbet Benson et al., "The Effect of Meditative Movement on Sleep Quality: A Systematic Review," *Sleep Medicine Reviews* 30 (December 17, 2015): 43–52, https://doi.org/10.1016/j.smrv.2015.12.001.
16. Upper airway resistance syndrome is another; unlike OSA, it often presents with less snoring, no gasping for air, and may be associated with low blood pressure.
17. Hartmut Schulz and Piero Salzarulo, "The Development of Sleep Medicine: A Historical Sketch," *Journal of Clinical Sleep Medicine* 12, no. 7 (July 14, 2016): 1041–52, https://doi.org/10.5664/jcsm.5946.
18. Marc L. Molendijk, Ouarda Bouachmir, Harriet Montagne, Laura Bowman, and Jan Dirk Blom, "The Incubus Phenomenon: Prevalence, Frequency and Risk Factors in Psychiatric Inpatients and University Undergraduates," *Fron-*

tiers in Psychiatry 13 (November 14, 2022): 1040769, https://doi.org/10.3389/fpsyt.2022.1040769.

19. Milo A Puhan, Alex Suarez, Christian Lo Cascio, Alfred Zahn, Markus Heitz, and Otto Braendli, "Didgeridoo Playing as Alternative Treatment for Obstructive Sleep Apnoea Syndrome: Randomised Controlled Trial," *BMJ* 332, no. 7536 (December 23, 2005): 266–70, https://doi.org/10.1136/bmj.38705.470590.55.
20. M. P. Hilton, J. O. Savage, B. Hunter, S. McDonald, C. Repanos, and R. Powell, "Singing Exercises Improve Sleepiness and Frequency of Snoring Among Snorers—A Randomised Controlled Trial," *International Journal of Otolaryngology and Head & Neck Surgery* 2, no. 3 (January 1, 2013): 97–102, https://doi.org/10.4236/ijohns.2013.23023.
21. Macario Camacho, Victor Certal, Jose Abdullatif, Soroush Zaghi, Chad M. Ruoff, Robson Capasso et al., "Myofunctional Therapy to Treat Obstructive Sleep Apnea: A Systematic Review and Meta-Analysis," *Sleep* 38, no. 5 (April 30, 2015): 669–75, https://doi.org/10.5665/sleep.4652.
22. Liaoyao Wang, Jia Xu, Yijun Zhan, and Jian Pei, "Acupuncture for Obstructive Sleep Apnea (OSA) in Adults: A Systematic Review and Meta-Analysis," *BioMed Research International* 2020, no. 1 (January 1, 2020): 6972327, https://doi.org/10.1155/2020/6972327.
23. Thomas D. Hurwitz, Mark W. Mahowald, Carlos H. Schenck, L. Janet, and Scott R. Bundlie, "A Retrospective Outcome Study and Review of Hypnosis as Treatment of Adults with Sleepwalking and Sleep Terror," *The Journal of Nervous and Mental Disease* 179, no. 4 (April 1, 1991): 228–33, https://doi.org/10.1097/00005053-199104000-00009.
24. Kazuhiko Fukuda, Akio Miyasita, Maki Inugami, and Kaneyoshi Ishihara, "High Prevalence of Isolated Sleep Paralysis: Kanashibari Phenomenon in Japan," *Sleep* 10, no. 3 (May 1, 1987): 279–86, https://doi.org/10.1093/sleep/10.3.279.

4. Transforming the Mind for Rest

1. Alan Watts, *The Way of Zen* (Vintage, 1999).
2. Thich Nhat Hanh, *Fear: Essential Wisdom for Getting Through the Storm* (HarperOne, 2012).
3. Hanh, *Fear*, 139.
4. Thich Nhat Hanh, *Being Peace* (Parallax Press, 2024).
5. Søren Kierkegaard, *The Concept of Anxiety: A Simple Psychologically Orienting Deliberation on the Dogmatic Issue of Hereditary Sin*, trans. Alastair Hannay (Princeton University Press, 1980).
6. Hanh, *Fear*.

7. Hanh, *Fear*, 39.
8. Pema Chödrön, *The Places That Scare You: A Guide to Fearlessness in Difficult Times* (Shambhala Publications, 2018).
9. Chödrön, *The Places That Scare You*, 52.
10. Hanh, *Fear*.

5. Dreams as the Window into the Unconscious

1. Chogyal Namkhai Norbu and Jamgon Mipham, *Buddhist Dream Yoga: Dzogchen and the Practice of Natural Light* (Shambhala Publications, 2025), xxvi.
2. Patrick McNamara, *The Neuroscience of Sleep and Dreams* (Cambridge University Press, 2023), 196–97. This theory was updated by Hobson in 2000 as the Activation-Input Source-Neuromodulation Model or AIM model of dreaming in which cortical activation in addition to brainstem activation is given great weight.
3. McNamara, *The Neuroscience of Sleep and Dreams*, 207–8.
4. Frederick L. Coolidge, *Evolutionary Neuropsychology: An Introduction to the Evolution of the Structures and Functions of the Human Brain* (Oxford University Press, 2020), 192.
5. McNamara, *The Neuroscience of Sleep and Dreams*, 208–10.
6. Antonio Zadra and Robert Stickgold, *When Brains Dream: Exploring the Science and Mystery of Sleep* (W. W. Norton & Co, 2021), 108–11.
7. Names and certain descriptors have been changed to preserve anonymity throughout the book.
8. McNamara, *The Neuroscience of Sleep and Dreams*, 185.
9. B. Alan Wallace and Brian Hodel, *Dreaming Yourself Awake: Lucid Dreaming and Tibetan Dream Yoga for Insight and Transformation* (Shambhala Publications, 2012), 32–33.
10. Larry Burk and Kathleen O'Keefe-Kanavos, *Dreams That Can Save Your Life: Early Warning Signs of Cancer and Other Diseases* (Findhorn Press, 2018).
11. Dbyaṅs-Can-Dga'-Ba'i-Blo-Gros, Lati Rinbochay, and Jeffrey Hopkins, *Death, Intermediate State, and Rebirth in Tibetan Buddhism* (Snow Lion, 1985).

6. Turning Air into Rest with Breathwork

1. Thich Nhat Hanh, *The Miracle of Mindfulness: An Introduction to the Practice of Meditation* (Beacon Press, 1999).
2. Jon Kabat-Zinn, *Wherever You Go, There You Are: Mindfulness Meditation in Everyday Life* (Hyperion, 2005), 13.
3. Pema Chödrön, *The Places That Scare You: A Guide to Fearlessness in Difficult Times* (Shambhala Publications, 2018).
4. Shirley Telles, Ram Kumar Gupta, Arti Yadav, Shivangi Pathak, and Ach-

arya Balkshrina, "Hemisphere Specific EEG Related to Alternate Nostril Yoga Breathing," *BMC Research Notes* 10, no. 1 (July 24, 2017): 306, https://doi.org/10.1186/s13104-017-2625-6.

5. Allison G. Harvey and Suzanna Payne, "The Management of Unwanted Pre-Sleep Thoughts in Insomnia: Distraction with Imagery Versus General Distraction," *Behaviour Research and Therapy* 40, no. 3 (March 1, 2002): 267–77, https://doi.org/10.1016/s0005-7967(01)00012-2.
6. Aayushi Khajuria, Nitesh Singh Malan, Rishabh Bajpai, Dimpy Kapoor, Ashish Mishra, Shivkumar Harti et al., "Investigating the Brain Activity Correlates of Humming Bee Sound During Bhramari Pranayama," *Annals of Indian Academy of Neurology* 26, no. 4 (July 1, 2023): 461–68, https://doi.org/10.4103/aian.aian_418_23.

7. Shadow Work and Emotional Healing

1. Julia Kristeva, *Strangers to Ourselves* (Columbia University Press, 1991).
2. Robert Louis Stevenson, *The Strange Case of Dr. Jekyll and Mr. Hyde and Other Tales of Terror* (Penguin Classics, 2003).
3. Robert Augustus Masters, *Bringing Your Shadow Out of the Dark: Breaking Free from the Hidden Forces That Drive You* (Sounds True, 2018), 48.

8. Sound Therapy and Silence

1. Daniel J. Levitin, *I Heard There Was a Secret Chord: Music as Medicine* (W. W. Norton & Company, 2024), 81–93.
2. Levitin, *I Heard There Was a Secret Chord*, 166.
3. Hertz is the measurement of how fast a sound wave is vibrating. Higher hertz numbers mean the sound is vibrating more times per second. Wavelength tells us how far apart those vibrations are. Together, they help define the pitch and quality of the sounds we hear.
4. Hwa-Ah-Ni Lee, Woo-Jin Lee, Seong-Uk Kim, Hyunji Kim, Minkyu Ahn, Jeonghui Kim et al., "Effect of Dynamic Binaural Beats on Sleep Quality: A Proof-of-Concept Study with Questionnaire and Biosignals," *SLEEP* 47, no. 10 (April 17, 2024), https://doi.org/10.1093/sleep/zsae097.
5. Kaho Akimoto, Ailing Hu, Takuji Yamaguchi, and Hiroyuki Kobayashi, "Effect of 528 Hz Music on the Endocrine System and Autonomic Nervous System," *Health* 10, no. 9 (January 1, 2018): 1159–70, https://doi.org/10.4236/health.2018.109088.
6. Dongrui Gao, Siyu Long, Hua Yang, Yobi Cheng, Sijia Guo, Yue Yu et al., "SWS Brain-Wave Music May Improve the Quality of Sleep: An EEG Study," *Frontiers in Neuroscience* 14 (February 11, 2020): 67, https://doi.org/10.3389/fnins.2020.00067.

7. Muse is a wearable EEG-powered "brain sensing headband" that monitors your brain-wave activity in real time, then translates that data into feedback (via sound cues and app prompts) to help improve focus, relaxation, and sleep.
8. Pico Iyer, *Aflame: Learning from Silence* (Penguin Group, 2025).

9. Harnessing the Power of Light and Dark

1. A. Roger Ekirch, *At Day's Close: Night in Times Past* (W. W. Norton & Company, 2005).
2. Wolfgang Schivelbusch, *Disenchanted Night: The Industrialization of Light in the Nineteenth Century* (University of California Press, 1995).
3. Timothy M. Brown, George C. Brainard, Christian Cajochen, Charles A. Czeisler, John P. Hanifin, Steven W. Lockley et al., "Recommendations for Daytime, Evening, and Nighttime Indoor Light Exposure to Best Support Physiology, Sleep, and Wakefulness in Healthy Adults," *PLoS Biology* 20, no. 3 (March 17, 2022): e3001571, https://doi.org/10.1371/journal.pbio.3001571.
4. Ivy C. Mason, Daniela Grimaldi, Kathryn J. Reid, Chloe D. Warlick, Roneil G. Malkani, Sabra M. Abbott et al., "Light Exposure During Sleep Impairs Cardiometabolic Function," *Proceedings of the National Academy of Sciences* 119, no. 12 (March 14, 2022): e2113290119, https://doi.org/10.1073/pnas.2113290119.
5. Anne-Marie Chang, Daniel Aeshbach, Jeanne F. Duffy, and Charles A. Czeisler, "Evening Use of Light-Emitting eReaders Negatively Affects Sleep, Circadian Timing, and Next-Morning Alertness," *Proceedings of the National Academy of Sciences* 112, no. 4 (December 22, 2014): 1232–37, https://doi.org/10.1073/pnas.1418490112.

10. Adjusting Your Diet to Support Sleep

1. Mark D. Miller, Craig Steinmaus, Mari S. Golub, Rosemary Castorina, Ruwan Thilakartne, Asa Bradman et al., "Potential Impacts of Synthetic Food Dyes on Activity and Attention in Children: A Review of the Human and Animal Evidence," *Environmental Health* 21, no. 1 (April 29, 2022): 45, https://doi.org/10.1186/s12940-022-00849-9.
2. Wolfgang Schivelbusch, *Tastes of Paradise: A Social History of Spices, Stimulants, and Intoxicants* (Vintage, 1993).
3. Hassan S. Dashti, Frank A. J. L. Scheer, Paul F. Jacques, Stefania Lamon-Fava, and Jose M. Ordovas, "Short Sleep Duration and Dietary Intake: Epidemiologic Evidence, Mechanisms, and Health Implications," *Advances in Nutrition* 6, no. 6 (November 1, 2015): 648–59, https://doi.org/10.3945/an.115.008623.

4. Stephanie M. Greer, Andrea N. Goldstein, and Matthew P. Walker, "The Impact of Sleep Deprivation on Food Desire in the Human Brain," *Nature Communications* 4, no. 1 (August 6, 2013): 2259, https://doi.org/10.1038/ncomms3259.
5. Matthew Walker, *Why We Sleep: Unlocking the Power of Sleep and Dreams* (Scribner, 2018), 177.
6. Ian M. Colrain, Christian L. Nicholas, and Fiona C. Baker, "Alcohol and the Sleeping Brain," *Handbook of Clinical Neurology* 125 (January 1, 2014): 415–31, https://doi.org/10.1016/b978-0-444-62619-6.00024-0.

11. Sleep as a Little Death

1. Pema Chödrön, *How We Live Is How We Die* (Shambhala Publications, 2022).
2. Chödrön, *How We Live Is How We Die*, 118.
3. Francis V. Tiso, *Rainbow Body and Resurrection: Spiritual Attainment, the Dissolution of the Material Body, and the Case of Khenpo A Chö* (North Atlantic Books, 2016), 24.
4. Sam Mauhay-Moore, "California Teen Lost Touch with Reality, Walked off Mount Whitney, Dad Says 'He Was in an Altered Mental State, and I Don't Know What Caused It,'" *SFGATE*, June 25, 2025, https://www.sfgate.com/bayarea/article/california-teen-hiker-coma-mount-whitney-20392404.php.

Afterword

1. Robert Pfaller, *Interpassivity: The Aesthetics of Delegated Enjoyment* (Incitements, 2017).
2. Slavoj Žižek, *The Plague of Fantasies* (Verso Books, 2009).
3. Oldis, D., Animating Dreams and Future Dream Recording, Poster presented at the 34th Annual Conference of the International Association for the Study of Dreams, 2017, Anaheim, CA.
4. T. Horikawa, M. Tamaki, Y. Miyawaki, and Y. Kamitani, "Neural Decoding of Visual Imagery During Sleep," *Science* 340, no. 6132 (April 4, 2013): 639–42, https://doi.org/10.1126/science.1234330.

Appendix B

1. Nancy Digdon and Amy Koble, "Effects of Constructive Worry, Imagery Distraction, and Gratitude Interventions on Sleep Quality: A Pilot Trial," *Applied Psychology: Health and Well-Being* 3, no. 2 (May 24, 2011): 193–206, https://doi.org/10.1111/j.1758-0854.2011.01049.x.

INDEX

ABOUT THE AUTHOR

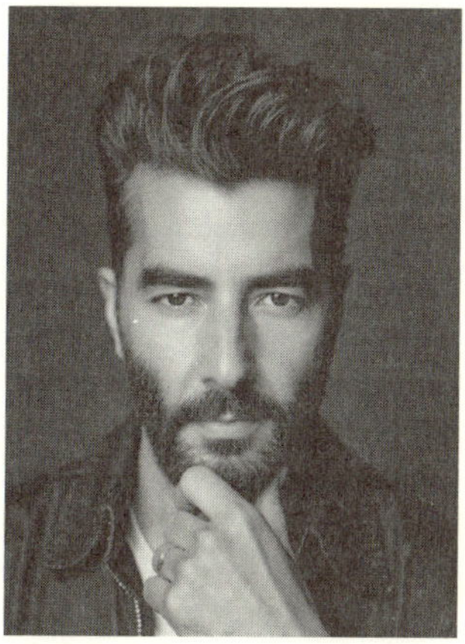

DR. PEDRAM NAVAB is a neurologist, sleep and integrative medicine specialist, and attorney whose work bridges medicine, law, and literature. He was educated at Brown University and completed a sleep medicine fellowship at Stanford. He is currently a sleep medicine consultant at the Hoag Voltmer Sleep Center in Newport Beach, California, where he is the vice chair of the Neurology and Psychiatry Department and treats insomnia and a variety of sleep disorders. He has served on the Advocacy and Public Safety Committees of the American Academy of Sleep Medicine and has lobbied for permanent standard time at the Capitol. He has been featured on *The Today Show* and in publications such as *Time, HuffPost, Salon,* and *Glamour*. In addition to his medical and legal work, Navab is a novelist whose fiction explores the psychological and surreal. *The Alchemy of Sleep* draws on his multidisciplinary background to offer a profound and original exploration of rest, dreams, and the unconscious mind.